John F. Kurtzke

Epidemiology of Cerebrovascular Disease

With 42 Figures

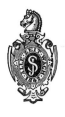

Springer-Verlag Berlin · Heidelberg · New York 1969

John F. Kurtzke, M. D.
Professor of Neurology and Professor of Community Medicine
and International Health, Georgetown University School of Medicine;
Chief, Neurology Service, Veterans Administration Hospital,
Washington, D.C.; Consultant in Neurology, U.S. Naval Hospital,
National Naval Medical Center, Bethesda, Md.

To my wife

Foreword

This work started out quite modestly as an investigation into the geographic distribution of cerebrovascular disease. But one question soon led to another and it just growed, like Topsy. In fact, it is hard to characterize precisely what this should be called. It is in part a Review of the Literature, in part a critique and reworking of other publications, and in part a standard view of stroke epidemiology in the more restricted sense of attack and mortality rates and distribution. Still the result would I hope provide a synthesis of the population features of stroke as they appear to me at this time — a highly individual interpretation of the "state of the art".

I have studiously avoided any survey of the history of cerebrovascular disease, and citations are for those of most recent vintage appropriate to the situation. Literature in this field continues to burgeon; my references end with the Fall of 1967. When counting noses we must have numbers, so the reader will find a massive compilation of tables. They are however necessary, especially since so many of my statements seem to fly in the face of current orthodoxy, whether lay or medical. With the data, one may decide for himself their validity. Insofar as possible tables have been placed in the appendix. Unless an author is directly quoted by me, all interpretations of his data are my own and he should be held blameless. Additionally, nothing in this work should be construed as representing the opinions or policy of the Veterans Administration, the Department of the Navy, or Georgetown University.

November 1, 1968   J. F. KURTZKE

Contents

List of Text Tables IX

List of Figures XI

List of Appendix Tables XIII

Chapter I. Epidemiology. Definitions and Methods 1
  Epidemiologic Methods. Case-Material Sources. Statistical Testing.
  References.

Chapter II. Definitions of Cerebrovascular Disease 8
  International Statistical Classification of CVD. Clinical Definitions.
  References.

Chapter III. On the Validity of Mortality Data 12
  (no subsections). References.

Chapter IV. General Features of Cerebral Vascular Disease 17
  Mortality Data. Incidence Data. Sex Ratios in CVD. References.

Chapter V. The Geographic Distribution of CVD 29
  Sweden. Norway. Denmark. Scandinavian Medical Facilities and CVD
  Distribution. Ireland. United States. References.

Chapter VI. CVD — Major Divisions and Subarachnoid Hemorrhage 47
  Relative Frequency of Types of CVD. Subarachnoid Hemorrhage —
  Mortality Data. SAH — Clinical Data. SAH — Aneurysm. SAH —
  AVM. SAH — Other. SAH — Integration. References

Chapter VII. Cerebral Hemorrhage and Thrombosis 60
  Cerebral Hemorrhage. Cerebral Thrombosis-Embolism. Autopsy Data
  in Thromboembolism. Clinical Components of Thromboembolism. Transient Ischemic Attacks. Sex Ratios in Thromboembolism. References.

Chapter VIII. Race and the Japan Story 69
  CVD in the American Negro. CVD in South Africa. CVD in Japan.
  The Dénouement. References.

Chapter IX. Factors Associated with CVD 81
  Hypertension. CAD and Arteriosclerosis. Serum Cholesterol and Lipids.
  Smoking. Other Associated Factors. References.

Chapter X. Changing Times and CVD 90
  SAH. Cerebral Hemorrhage. Cerebral Thrombosis. References.

Chapter XI. The Course of CVD 96
  All CVD. SAH. Cerebral Hemorrhage. Cerebral Thrombosis. References.

Chapter XII. CVD — Comments and Conclusions 106
    A Suggested Code for CVD. Geographic Distribution of CVD. Sex Ratios.
    Race and CVD. Related Factors. Stroke, Age, and Implications. Refe-
    rences.

Chapter XIII. Summary by Chapters 113

References 125

Appendix 142

Subject Index 195

List of Text Tables

IV—1.   Age adjusted annual mortality rates for CVD in 18 countries ...   17
IV—2.   CVD as proportion of deaths in elderly in Eire and Scandinavia   23
IV—3.   Sex ratios from age specific mortality rates for CVD   28
V—1.   Distribution of CVD deaths in Sweden (1933 and 1960)   30
V—2.   Distribution of CVD deaths in Norway (1946)   33
V—3.   Distribution of CVD in Denmark (1950 and 1960)   34
V—4.   Age specific distributions of CVD in Denmark (1961)   37
V—5.   Correlations of CVD and medical facilities in Scandinavia   37
V—6.   Distribution of CVD deaths in Ireland (1951—1955)   39
V—7.   Distribution of CVD deaths in United States (1959—1961)   40
V—8.   Correlations of CVD and physicians in United States   41
VI—1.   Percentage frequencies for types of CVD   48
VI—2.   Age frequencies of SAH vs. other CVD deaths   49
VI—3.   Major causes of SAH   53
VI—4.   Distributions by sex and site for single aneurysms   55
VII—1. Age specific annual incidence rates for cerebral thrombosis   62
VII—2. Age frequencies for carotid vs. vertebrobasilar occlusions   64
VII—3. Distributions by type and site for Cb thrombosis-embolism   65
VII—4. Proportions for cerebral embolism to thrombosis   65
VII—5. Distributions by sex and site for TIA   66
VII—6. Various characteristics of TIA   67
VIII—1. CVD mortality rates by type, race, and sex in Memphis   69
VIII—2. Age specific CVD mortality rates by race and sex in U.S.A. (1950)   72
VIII—3. Mortality rates for CVD, CA, heart disease in Japan (1900—1960)   75
VIII—4. CVD as proportion of deaths in the elderly in Japan (1910, 1962)   78
VIII—5. CVD deaths in Japanese adult population sample (1962—1963)   78
VIII—6. CVD in Hisayama, Japan from population survey (1961—1965)   79
XI—1.   Cumulative case-fatality rates for all CVD by age   97
XI—2.   Major causes and course of SAH   99
XI—3.   Frequency of intracerebral hemorrhage and death in SAH by type   99
XI—4.   Frequency of early deaths by site of aneurysm   100
XI—5.   Cumulative case-fatality rates for cerebral thrombosis and hemor-
        rhage   103

List of Figures

IV–1.   Age specific annual mortality rates for CVD in U.S. and England   18

IV–2.   Age specific annual mortality rates for CVD in Denmark   19

IV–3.   Age specific annual mortality rates for CVD in Norway, Sweden, and Ireland   20

IV–4.   Age specific annual mortality rates for CVD in Canada   21

IV–5.   Age specific annual mortality rates for CVD in San Francisco . . .   22

IV–6.   Age frequency distribution for CVD, incidence and mortality data   24

IV–7.   Age specific annual incidence rates for CVD in Connecticut and Minnesota   25

IV–8.   Age specific annual incidence rates for CVD in Carlisle, Missouri, and England   26

IV–9.   Age frequency distribution for CVD cases in Goulburn, Australia   27

V–1.   Distribution of urban CVD deaths by county in Sweden (1933) . .   31

V–2.   Distribution of CVD deaths by county in Norway (1946) and Sweden (1960) with population 60 and over as base   32

V–3.   Distribution of CVD deaths by county in Sweden (1960), total population   33

V–4.   Distribution of "CVD" deaths in Denmark (1950) in percentiles of mean   34

V–5.   Distribution of "CVD" deaths in Denmark (1950) in χ-square ranges   35

V–6.   Distribution of CVD deaths in Denmark (1960) in percentiles of mean   35

V–7.   Distribution of CVD deaths in Denmark (1960) in χ-square ranges   36

V–8.   Distribution of CVD deaths by county in Eire (1951—1955)   38

V–9.   Distribution of white male CVD deaths by state in USA (1959 to 1961)   42

V–10.   Distribution of white female CVD deaths by state in USA (1959 to 1961)   43

V–11.   Distribution of physicians by state in USA (1962)   44

V–12.   Correlation of CVD and physician distributions in USA   45

V–13.   Correlation of CVD and physician distributions in Scandinavia . .   46

VI–1.   Age frequency for SAH vs. other CVD deaths in England   50

VI–2.   Age specific annual mortality rates for SAH and other CVD in
Denmark   51

VI–3.   Age specific annual mortality rates for SAH in the Netherlands..   52

VI–4.   Age frequency for SAH with aneurysm   54

VI–5.   Age frequency for SAH, brain tumor, and other CVD...........   54

VI–6.   Age frequency for AVM   55

VI–7.   Age frequency for idiopathic SAH   56

VI–8.   SAH — cause and effect...................................   58

VII–1. Age specific annual mortality rates for hemorrhage, thrombosis,
and "other" CVD in Denmark (1956—1960)   61

VIII–1. Age specific annual mortality rates for CVD in US Negroes......   70

VIII–2. as above, corrected for population bias......................   72

VIII–3. Age specific annual mortality rates for CVD by race in South Africa   73

VIII–4. Age specific annual mortality rates for CVD in Japan (1910)   74

VIII–5. Age specific annual mortality rates for CVD in Japan (1950)   76

VIII–6. Age specific annual mortality rates for CVD in Japan (1962)   77

XI–1.   Cumulative case-fatality rates for CVD by age at ictus..........   98

XI–2.   Cumulative case-fatality rates for SAH by cause   98

XI–3.   Cumulative case-fatality rates for Cb H, Cb Thr-Emb, and "other"
CVD   102

XII–1. Age frequency for occlusions, encephalomalacia, and autopsies...   110

XII–2. Age specific annual mortality rates for all deaths in England (1851
and 1951) vs. CVD rates in USA — England   111

List of Appendix Tables

IV—a—1.   Age specific annual mortality rates for CVD, USA and England-Wales 142
IV—a—2.   Population and CVD deaths by age and sex in Denmark (1950) 142
IV—a—3.   CVD deaths as percentage of total deaths in Denmark (1950) 143
IV—a—4.   CVD deaths as in IV—a—3 in Sweden (1956—1960) 143
IV—a—5.   Age specific annual mortality rates for CVD in Denmark (1950) 144
IV—a—6.   as above, Denmark (1956) 144
IV—a—7.   as above, Denmark (1960) 144
IV—a—8.   as above, Norway (1946) 145
IV—a—9.   as above, Sweden (1933)................................ 145
IV—a—10.   as above, Sweden (1960)................................ 145
IV—a—11.   as above, Ireland (1951) 146
IV—a—12.   as above, Canada (1960—1964) 146
IV—a—13.   as above, San Francisco (1962—1964) 147
IV—a—14.   Age frequency CVD cases in Connecticut survey 147
IV—a—15.   Age specific annual incidence rates for CVD in Connecticut and Minnesota 147
IV—a—16.   as above (IV—a—15) in several US surveys 148
IV—a—17.   as above, in Carlisle, England and in Missouri 148
IV—a—18.   Age frequency CVD cases in Goulburn, Australia 149
IV—a—19.   as in IV—a—15, in British general practices 149
IV—a—20.   as in IV—a—15, hospital cases in Frederiksberg, Denmark ... 149
IV—a—21.   Sex ratios in CVD from mortality statistics 150
IV—a—22.   Sex ratios in CVD from hospital series and population surveys 150
V—a—1.   Distribution CVD deaths by county in Norway (1946), total population 151
V—a—2.   same, population age 60 and over 151
V—a—3.   Distribution of physicians by county in Norway (1946) 152
V—a—4.   Distribution of hospital facilities in Norway (1946—1948) .. 153
V—a—5.   Distribution urban CVD deaths by county in Sweden (1933), with urban population age 60 and over 154
V—a—6.   Distribution CVD deaths by county in Sweden (1960), total population 155
V—a—7.   Distribution CVD deaths in Sweden (1960), population 60 and over 156
V—a—8.   Distribution physicians and hospitals in Sweden (1933) 157
V—a—9.   Distribution of urban physicians in Sweden (1933) 158
V—a—10.   Distribution of "CVD" deaths by county in Denmark (1950), total population.. 159
V—a—11.   same, population 60 and over 160

V–a–12.   Distribution of physicians by county in Denmark (1950) ...   161
V–a–13.   Distribution of specialists and hospital facilities in Denmark
          (1950)   126
V–a–14.   Distribution of CVD deaths by county in Denmark (1960),
          total population   163
V–a–15.   same, population 60 and over............................   164
V–a–16.   Frequency distributions of CVD deaths in Denmark (1960)
          by age, sex, and area   165
V–a–17.   Correlations of medical facilities in Sweden (1933)   165
V–a–18.   Distribution of CVD deaths by county in Eire (1951—1955)   169
V–a–19.   Distribution by state of physicians in USA (1962)   167
V–a–20.   Distribution of CVD deaths in Denmark (1961) by region,
          cases and population   168
VI–a–1.   Age-adjusted average annual mortality rates for types of
          CVD in 18 countries (1951—1958).......................   168
VI–a–2.   Cumulative frequency percentages by age for SAH and all
          other CVD deaths in Denmark (1956—1960)   169
VI–a–3.   Annual age specific mortality rates for SAH and rest of CVD
          in Denmark   170
VI–a–4.   Annual age specific mortality rates for SAH in the Nether-
          lands (1950—1954 and 1958—1962)   171
VI–a–5.   Age frequencies by major cause of SAH   171
VI–a–6.   Age frequencies for aneurysm and brain tumor in London ...   172
VI–a–7.   Frequencies by site and sex for single aneurysms   172
VI–a–8.   Age frequencies for AVM from Cooperative Study..........   173
VI–a–9.   Age frequencies for AVM from Mayo Clinic   173
VI–a–10. Age frequencies for SAH with HT and/or AS..............   173
VI–a–11. Age frequencies for idiopathic SAH   174
VI–a–12. Sex ratios for SAH   174
VI–a–13. Sex ratios from age specific mortality rates for SAH in Den-
          mark   174
VII–a–1. Age frequencies by type of CVD deaths in Denmark (1956
          to 1960)   175
VII–a–2. Age specific annual mortality rates by type of CVD in Den-
          mark   176
VII–a–3. Age frequencies for Cb thrombosis and hemorrhage cases from
          US population surveys   176
VII–a–4. Age specific annual mortality rates for Cb hemorrhage deaths
          in hospital in Göteborg, Sweden (1948—1949 and 1960—1961)   177
VII–a–5. Age specific annual incidence rates for Cb hemorrhage cases
          from US population surveys   177
VII–a–6. Sex ratios in Cb hemorrhage   177
VII–a–7. Sex ratios in Cb hemorrhage from age specific mortality rates
          in Denmark (1956—1960)   178
VII–a–8. Age frequencies for recent encephalomalacia in New Orleans   178
VII–a–9. Age specific rates (per autopsies) for intracranial occlusions,
          N. Y.   178

VII—a—10. Age frequencies for complicated arteriosclerosis and ence-
           phalomalacia in New Orleans 179
VII—a—11. Frequencies by site of thromboembolic occlusions, in Oslo 179
VII—a—12. Frequencies by site of encephalomalacia in New York 180
VII—a—13. Comparison of age distributions in carotid and vertebrobasilar
           lesions 180
VII—a—14. Frequencies of TIA by sex, age, and site, in London 180
VII—a—15. Sex ratios for Cb thrombosis-embolism 181
VII—a—16. Sex ratios for thrombosis-embolism and "other" CVD from
           age specific mortality rates in Denmark (1956—1960) 181
VII—a—17. Sex ratios for subdivisions of Cb thrombosis-embolism 182
VIII—a—1. Age specific annual mortality rates for CVD in non-whites,
           US (1960) 182
VIII—a—2. as above, corrected for population bias.................. 183
VIII—a—3. Age specific annual mortality rates for CVD by race in South
           Africa (1954—1958) 183
VIII—a—4. CVD hospital deaths in Johannesburg, South Africa (to 1960) 184
VIII—a—5. Age specific annual mortality rates for CVD in Japan (1910) 184
VIII—a—6. Population and Cb hemorrhage deaths in Japan (1950, 1962) 185
VIII—a—7. Age specific annual mortality rates for Cb hemorrhage in
           Japan (1950, 1962) 186
VIII—a—8. as above, for SAH................................... 187
VIII—a—9. as above, for Cb thrombosis-embolism 188
VIII—a—10. as above, for "other" CVD 189
VIII—a—11. as above, for 332 plus 334 ISC rubrics 190
VIII—a—12. as above, for all CVD (330 to 334) 191
VIII—a—13. Diagnostic revisions with time for CVD in the first two years
           of the Hisayama study................................ 191
XI—a—1.   Distribution of CVD deaths by age and interval, from Con-
           necticut.. 192
XI—a—2.   Cumulative case-fatality rates for first SAH by cause 192
XI—a—3.   Distribution of CVD deaths by type and interval, from Con-
           necticut.. 193
XI—a—4.   Comparison of course, carotid and vertebrobasilar thrombosis 193
XII—a—1.   Age frequencies for occlusions, encephalomalacia, and autop-
           sies 194
XII—a—2.   Age specific mortality rates for all deaths in England (1851,
           1951) 194

Chapter I

Epidemiology

Definition and Methods

The narrow construct of epidemiology as pertaining to epidemics has been broadened by its proper definition as the discourse or study (lógos) upon (epi) people (dēmos). Though by custom limited to the disorders to which the flesh is heir, one must also consider in this context the normal to recognize deviations therefrom. Thus epidemiology is concerned with the occurrence and course of disease within populations. It is diagnosis and prognosis of groups rather than individuals, the signs and symptoms being those features which differentiate the patient from his unaffected peer. PAUL's definition is that epidemiology is the field "concerned with measurements of the circumstances under which diseases occur, where diseases tend to flourish, and where they do not" (p. 4). In other words it is the study of the natural history of disease — including our attempts to alter the course by varied therapeutic measures. In this context epidemiology could be considered the basic science of clinical medicine.

In defining a new disease, it is the similarities in symptoms among patients which lead us to feel that we are dealing with a syndrome distinct from other disease-states. Common features from the physical examination and the laboratory confirm us in this belief, and detailed study of associated factors permits us (when successful) to define the cause of this-now-disease. Knowledge of cause permits us to devise a treatment, whose efficacy is determined by its alteration of the natural course of the illness. Note in all these steps we are considering groups, not individuals. The features that patients have in common permit us to develop a body of knowledge, the science of medicine, while their unalterable individualities demand of us an equally important skill, the art of medicine.

The concepts of etiology — again from PAUL — include the seed and the soil, as taken from the Gospel according to Matthew, and the climate. The seed is the Aristotelian essential cause, that without which the disease cannot occur; whether it be the tubercle bacillus, methanol, or a blow on the head, it is the etiologic agent. The soil is the host, which may be fertile or fallow for the seed dependent upon innate, chiefly genetic, factors; and the climate is "the environment to which seed and soil are exposed". This environment includes the general milieu, the macro-climate — and geographic pathology is one branch of epidemiology. It also includes the individual microclimate which is the resultant of one's past experiences and current physical, mental, and socioeconomic situation.

The epidemiologic process attempts to answer who is afflicted with our disease (the what), as well as when and where does this occur, and hopefully why. The question of "what", that is clinical diagnosis, is basic to all epidemiologic study. This is a matter influenced by many factors, such as current nomenclature, diagnostic fashions, medical standards, the frequency of the disease, the presence of pathognomonic physical signs, and the need for, or possibility of, laboratory confirmation. Thus certain diseases such as amyotrophic lateral sclerosis when diagnosed are usually correctly labeled, whereas others as chronic bronchitis or multiple sclerosis are more subject to variability. Like the existence of noise when the tree falls in a deserted forest, there is no disease until it is diagnosed. Therefore areas of grossly inadequate medical facilities are not amenable to epidemiologic inquiry without special effort.

Epidemiologic Methods

The first question asked about our disease, after diagnosis, is how common it is. More precisely, we ask how many cases are present at one time in our study population (the *prevalence rate* of the disease), and how many new cases of the disease occur in a unit time (the *incidence rate* of the disease). For chronic diseases, incidence (rate) times duration equals prevalence (rate). Note the denominator is the study population, or "population at risk". This is the defined group under observation, and may be the entirety of a town or a nation, or the employees of a company, or the veterans who survived a war. Depending on the disease and the questions asked, it is often more economical to concentrate on but a segment of the population, as delimited by age, race, sex, or other criteria. As we get further away from the general population for the denominator though, there is a risk that our conclusions or observations may not be properly subject to generalization. Prevalence and incidence rates are customarily expressed as ratios with convenient unit populations, such as cases per 100,000 population, or per 1000 population. Age-specific rates are expressed in similar fashion but with both numerator and denominator referring to a given age, such as age 10 to 14, or age 60 and over. There are also methods to overcome differences in age structure among different populations, by reconstituting the series as if the study population ages were the same as the standard; these are called "age-adjusted" rates.

Prevalence and incidence rates are the optimal measures to define disease frequency. Another common ratio of value is the *mortality rate*. This rate arises from the number of patients dying of a disease in a given population in a unit time, and, like an incidence rate, is ordinarily expressed as cases per 100,000 population per year. Again age- (and sex- and race-) specific rates can be used. The *case-fatality rate* on the other hand defines the frequency of death among the afflicted. If 40 patients die out of 100 with tuberculous meningitis in one year, the case-fatality rate is 40%, while if these 40 were part of a community of 10 million people, the annual mortality rate for this disease would be 0.4 per 100,000 population.

From a comparison of rates, whether prevalence, incidence, or mortality, we can define the geographic distribution of disease either among countries or within parts of a land. Before considering this in more detail, it would be advisable to ask how we find the cases for the numerators in question.

Case Material Sources

As previously mentioned, for our purposes a disease must be diagnosed to exist Ordinarily this means a physician is the intermediary between the individual with his disorder and his final allocation as a "case" for one of our population rates. Early studies of disease, and indeed those from which many of our illnesses have been demarcated, are simply a result of the physician relating his own experience, having suitably classified his material. While this is still an epidemiologic resource in unique situations, for most purposes the *office practice* as input has been supplanted. One use of such material will be considered though in later chapters.

Hospital series, that is records from hospitals and clinics, have been a valuable source of material properly considered epidemiologic, as well as the major basis for our current thinking in medical practice. It is with these data that we have defined most modern diseases and their treatment, and their usefulness requires little comment. They are however subject to serious bias. The presence of a patient in a hospital is the resultant of special facilities available there vs. elsewhere, special interests or skills of the staff, socioeconomic factors, space available, and the general culture which helps or hinders one to seek hospitalization for his disease. All these provide a sieve with holes of unknown size through which diseased patients are filtered. Further, those with the disease in a hospital are most often that undefinable fraction of the whole diseased group who do poorly. However, where a single hospital services an entire community, where the disease requires hospital diagnosis or treatment, and where the medical care for the disorder is not limited by social factors, then the data from hospital series can provide a useful epidemiologic resource. Especially from state-oriented medical care systems of high professional levels, such as in Scandinavia, a great deal of important information is available from hospital records. The appropriate translation of hospital data to a population-based rate will therefore be very much dependent upon the nature of the illness and the locale of the study.

Mortality statistics have certain marked advantages in establishing the frequency of a disease. In advanced cultures, death is an event that does not pass unnoticed, and laws require a reason for demise. The underlying cause of death is supposed to be regularly and uniformly coded according to the same rules in most lands, and this material is routinely published. There is the real benefit also that a case will be listed only once, the merit of which will be appreciated by any one who has searched hospital files. Mortality data will be considered more extensively in the next two chapters, but some of the major defects of this material can be noted here.

One drawback is that only one disease is allowed per person as the "underlying cause of death". Current efforts at retrieval of "associated diseases" could correct this to some extent, but these do not form the corpus of available statistics, whose prime asset is just that, that they are available. In this country very few deaths result in autopsies; thus the "underlying cause of death" is usually a clinical diagnosis. Therefore ease of recognition is an important feature in assessing mortality data. The case-fatality rate is obviously important; one would not seek to study coryza from death certificates. Diseases which are steadily progressive or rapidly fatal will generally be listed, whereas those which are indolent or remitting will often be omitted. Where the case-fatality rate is not 100%, we must also wonder how representative of the diseased are those who die.

Certain diseases are reportable as morbidity statistics in most nations, being acute contagious ills in general. None of these are in our sphere of current interest.

1*

Population surveys constitute the best yet most expensive and time consuming epidemiologic resource. They fall into two general categories, which might be called the "Assyrian" and the "in-law", which are appropriate respectively for unusual and common diseases. For the rare disorders, a concerted effort is made to identify those individuals with the illness or illnesses in a short period of time. "The Assyrian came down like a wolf on the fold." The prevalence or incidence study in such instances is performed by identifying a population, and then using all available resources to obtain a list of potential cases of the disease to be studied, including hospital and physicians' records, disability and insurance files, and rolls of special lay groups. Then the original roster is screened for the appropriate residence and a judgment made, with defined criteria, as to the correctness of the diagnosis. Obviously there can be no more cases included than were recognized in the first instance, a source of error very difficult to estimate. Whether the cases then are each examined or diagnosis made from records will be a function of the size of the study and the time available. This type of approach can also be used for direct evalution of an entire population but with limited goals, as, for example, the recording of blood pressure or visual acuity, or screening for diabetes or pulmonary disease.

The optimal population surveys are long-term undertakings wherein an entire community, *in toto* or of a given age, is kept under medical surveillance for a considerable period of time. They are reminiscent of the in-law who comes for a visit, pokes about the closets, and rearranges the furniture, until we wonder when, if ever, the visit will end. In this country the classic study of this nature is that from Framingham, Massachusetts, which will be considered *in extenso* below. Several communities in England have been similarly studied, and on both sides of the ocean there have been prospective surveys of specific groups (physicians, college graduates, veterans), with more or less limited goals. To be appropriate for such consideration the area in question has to be restricted in size and in migration. The population, and the physicians and hospitals, must cooperate fully. The major drawback of this approach is the necessary reliance upon a small number of cases to be expected, even after some years of work. And here too the goals must be limited since we cannot study *all* diseases. There is also the question of how representative of the disease *or* the population might be the data from one small region, and some consideration need be paid to the interaction of the survey team and the populace.

Although not generally considered epidemiologic works, there have been a number of cooperative studies, usually oriented toward therapy, wherein cases are provided from geographically scattered regions. Keeping in mind that large numbers do not prevent the bias of hospital series from appearing, still some of these works do provide an additional source of material worthy of assessment.

The natural history or course of the disease and the presence of associated factors can only be ascertained directly from population surveys or from hospital series. A unique subsection of hospital series is that represented by autopsy material. While there are a number of ways to consider the course of disease, the simplest is the case-fatality rate with time. This seems more understandable to most physicians than life-table analyses. Chronic disability is also a factor of obvious import in the course, but will not be a topic in this paper. In like fashion, the assessment of the efficacy of various modes of treatment is not here under consideration, but will be touched upon tangentially in some instances.

Statistical Testing

The essence of all science is measurement, and the essence of measurement is variability. Simply put, properly applied statistical tests give us some idea how confident we can be in the numbers we have at hand, be they prevalence rates or operative deaths. If we are comparing two (or more) sets of data, they give us some estimate of the chances that the sets do indeed differ. This last is usually expressed as a rejection of the null hypothesis that there is no difference between the sets at a given probability level. "Significant differences" though never tell us *why* the differences are present; it is the design of a properly-conducted experiment which permits us to reach the desired conclusion when such differences appear with our data. This is the basic reason behind random allocation and double-blind procedures in trials of therapy.

In epidemiologic works we very seldom attain the status of an "experiment", where, when results differ significantly, we can safely conclude (usually) that *either* a rare event has occurred, *or* the series are truly different. Most epidemiologic studies are "surveys" (see MAINLAND [1963] for discussions to this point). When their results differ, we conclude *either* a rare event has occurred, *or* the series are truly different, *or* there is hidden bias and the series were not truly comparable to start with.

One useful and instructive tool with frequency data is the calculation of confidence limits; they could be called "lack of confidence" limits, since they provide in general a sort of "minimum error" to be expected *if* the study were perfect in all respects. Their chief value may lie in the sobering influence they can have when one attempts to generalize from his data. The 95% confidence limits of a rate can be loosely considered as defining the interval within which the "true" rate for the parent population will lie 19 times out of 20, *if* the study represents a random sample of its theoretical population. For percentages (as in case-fatality rates) there are published tables which provide these limits. For prevalence or mortality rates, the confidence limits can be calculated by considering the cases to be distributed in what is called a Poisson series, which has the unique characteristic that the variance equals the mean, and in most instances the 95% confidence limits can be approximated from $x \pm 2\sqrt{x}$, where x is the number of cases providing the prevalence rate. For example, 25 cases in 50,000 population gives a rate of 50 per 100,000. The approximate 95% confidence limits are obtained from $25 \pm 2\sqrt{25}$, or 15 to 35 cases in 50,000, which give confidence limits of 30 to 70 per 100,000 for our observed rate of 50. For more precision, corrections for asymmetry can be used. More details are published on this and the following methods [KURTZKE, 1966 (4)], and of course are available in standard statistical texts. The ones listed in the references for this chapter are those used for the present work.

The chi-square contigency test may well be the most widely used statistical method, at least by non-statisticians. It is useful for comparing distributions, be they locations of aneurysms, treatment results, or ages of patients. In prevalence surveys it can be used to compare geographic distributions within parts of a survey region to determine whether there is a deviation from homogeneity. For this last, we calculate for each area the number of cases expected if all areas had the same prevalence or mortality rate. The square of the difference between the observed and expected numbers of cases divided by the expected number provides a value which is one component of the total χ-square, which in turn is the sum of such values from all areas. The formula thus is $\chi^2 = \Sigma\,(O-E)^2/E$. The significance of the χ-square statistic is found from appropriate tables, and, should it lead to a rejection of the null hypothesis of homogeneity at the 1% level ($P < 0.01$), then we conclude the distribution is not homogeneous. If the deviations are also large*, and if the high-frequency areas tend to form a cluster rather than being scattered throughout the land, it would then seem reasonable to conclude that there is an essential dependence of the disease upon the presence of a similarly-distributed environmental agent. With proper precautions this last conclusion could lead to the definition of our disease as one of an acquired exogenous nature. Note the three provisos: significant deviation from homogeneity; individual deviations which are large; and deviations which are patterned to form clusters or foci. To this must be added the ever present proviso of epidemiologic surveys — that there may be hidden bias.

The individual value of $(O-E)^2/E$ for any one geographic unit may be considered an approximate χ-square (χ_a^2) for this unit versus the mean or versus all other areas combined, and such values above 4.0 will usually be "significantly" different from the mean ($P < 0.05$). Use of these values rather than the prevalence or mortality rates to map out our units is preferable when the rates are based on rather small numbers.

In very common diseases — and this could well include strokes — the χ-square test for homogeneity may well result in "highly significant" values simply because the numbers are so large. For example, a 10% variation when 400 cases are expected gives a χ_a^2 value of 4.0. If all units were of this size and had no more than this degree of variation the total χ^2 value would be "significantly" high. This is analogous to differences between means of 40.0 and 40.5, which could be statistically "significant" if the numbers were large enough, but would hardly be considered of any biologic import. Therefore, in order to assess the geographic distributions of cerebrovascular diseases, it was decided a priori to pay more attention to the degree of variation and the presence of clustering than to the formal χ-square results.

A search for associated factors is a major part of our inquiry into disease. Statistical tests of correlation are generally of two kinds, the most common being the Pearsonian product-moment coefficient of correlation (FISHER, 1958, p. 183) or its related factor the linear regression coefficient. These are "parametric" tests, that is, based upon a theoretical distribution whose population parameters (chiefly the mean and standard deviation) have defined values and relationships. Note that statistically a "population" is an abstraction like a line or a circle, and epidemio-

---

* By "large" deviations I consider several units at least should be well beyond 25% of the mean rate (outside 75% to 125% of the mean). "Several units" would mean some $1/5$ of all units tested.

logically a "population" (at risk) is a real entity, and in both instances the term has meaning beyond general usage. The theoretical distribution underlying the Pearson coefficient is the Gaussian or "normal" distribution.

Since there is often a question whether our epidemiologic material follows a Gaussian curve, it may be preferable to use "non-parametric" tests of association, of which the best one for use when seeking roughly linear correlations is the Spearman coefficient of correlation (SIEGEL, 1956, p. 202). This is a rank-order test for comparing two distributions. If all units have the same rank in each distribution, the correlation will be + 1.00; the greater the differences in ranks, the lower will be the (positive) correlation coefficient. The formula is

$$r = 1 - \frac{6 \Sigma D^2}{N^3 - N}$$

where D is the difference in ranks for each unit, and N is the number of units.

Just as "significant differences" never tell us *why* our series differ, neither does a "significant association" tell us why they appear to be related. The old example is of the man who became drunk on vodka and tonic, gin and tonic, and rum and tonic; so he gave up tonic. We are especially uncertain about correlations over time. In the last 50 years there is a direct relationship between the price of whiskey and medical fees; there is also a relationship between deaths from bronchogenic carcinoma and the number of medical school graduates. While these examples are obvious, some others may not be so, such as a declining death rate from hypertension and from cerebral hemorrhage.

References

(note: references are cited throughout according to first author)

General epidemiology	Statistics	Specific epidemiology
BEHREND 28	ARKIN 17	CLEMMENSEN 57
DOLL 82	FISHER, R. A. 107—109	DREYER 85, 86
FLETCHER 111	HILL 152	GOLDBERG 125
FRANCIS 115	KURTZKE 193	HAENSZEL 137
GOLDSCHMIDT 126	MAINLAND 211—212	KNOWLER 179
MAY 225, 226	PETERS 293	KRUEGER 183, 184
McDONOUGH 229	SIEGEL 324	KURLAND 187
PAUL 284	SNEDECOR 331	KURTZKE 189—194
PEMBERTON 289	TATE 351	LOGAN 207
TAYLOR 358	YULE 408	NEEL 266
WITTS 389		OLSON 274
		SNOW 332

CHAPTER II

Definitions of Cerebrovascular Disease

As we noted, the prerequisite in studying a disease is its definition. Cerebrovascular disease (CVD) can be classified from the location of the vascular or the cerebral lesion, the nature of the insult, or the cause of the disease. A quite exhaustive categorization of "stroke" has been accomplished by the ad hoc Committee of the Academy of Neurology and published as a supplement in Neurology in 1958. While certainly all-inclusive, its very complexity prevents its application to epidemiologic works, where simplicity must at times take precedence over accuracy. The Committee nomenclature too included both clinical and pathologic criteria in diagnosis, which further limits its applicability.

The basic framework for diagnostic categories of cerebrovascular disease must be that utilized for mortality data. This can then be elaborated when we consider hospital and population series.

International Statistical Classification of CVD

The World Health Organization has published a manual of the International Statistical Classification (ISC) of Diseases, Injuries, and Causes of Death, the most recent (1957) containing the Seventh Revision of 1955.

In 1855 the International Statistical Congress at Paris adopted a list of 139 rubrics for the classification of disease and injury, which, with modifications, was the sole international method of classification for the rest of the century, though never universally adopted. The Bertillon Classification of Causes of Death supplanted this in 1893, and, with amendments, was in use as the International List of Causes of Death in the early part of this century. The Fifth revision of the International List in 1938 was in three parts: a detailed list of 200 titles, an intermediate list of 87, and an abridged list of 44. The International Conference for the Sixth Revision of the International Lists of Diseases and Causes of Death met in Paris in 1948 and approved the basic format currently in use, the modifications at the Seventh Revision being quite minor.

The Detailed List consists of 3-digit numbers representing 612 categories of diseases and deaths, 153 categories of causes of injury, and 189 categories of the nature of injuries. In the Tabular List of Inclusions and Four-digit Subcategories more detailed coding is available. There are also several summary lists: "A" is an intermediate list of 150 causes for tabulation of morbidity and mortality; "B" is an abbreviated list of 50 causes of death.

Vascular lesions affecting the central nervous system carry the rubrics 330 through 334. Traumatic lesions are specifically excluded. For morbidity classification *only*, the late sequelae of strokes are not included, but are rather classed under No. 352. The ISC divisions of CVD deaths are:

330 subarachnoid hemorrhage,
331 cerebral hemorrhage,
332 cerebral embolism and thrombosis,
333 spasm of cerebral arteries,
334 other and ill-defined vascular lesions affecting central nervous system.
Each category has a list of official equivalent terms for inclusion under that rubric, which shall be noted here, since there are considerable differences of opinion on some of these terms.

Subarachnoid hemorrhage (SAH) includes "meningeal hemorrhage; ruptured (congenital) cerebral aneurysm; and subarachnoid hemorrhage."

Arteriovenous malformations (if diagnosed) should not appear as a cause of death under 330, but rather under No. 223, even if they bled. This specific item is generally unretrievable from routine statistics.

Cerebral hemorrhage (Cb H) includes "apoplexy, hemorrhagic (stroke); rupture of blood vessel in the brain; subdural hematoma, not due to trauma"; and hemorrhage of various parts of the cranial cavity with or without mention of arterial hypertension or arteriosclerosis (the parts are listed).

One warning here is that "stroke" or "apoplexy" unqualified *could* be (and has been) erroneously included here, rather than under the proper No. 334.

Cerebral embolism and thrombosis (Cb thr-emb) includes various equivalents of cerebral or cerebellar "softening, thrombosis, embolism, or necrosis". "Thrombotic: apoplexy or brain softening"; and "embolic: apoplexy, paralysis, hemiplegia, or brain softening", are all specific equivalents.

From the clinical viewpoint, it would have been preferable to have separated embolism from thrombosis, though this is not always clinically possible. Another warning is that with earlier standards of official nomenclature, the entirety of cerebrovascular disease was usually referred to as "cerebral apoplexy" or "cerebral hemorrhage" (or literal translations of same). Thus a decline in cerebral hemorrhage with time could be little more than a reflection of coding rules.

Spasm of cerebral arteries is a remnant of early thinking in cerebrovascular disease. In recent figures it accounts for perhaps 1 in 30,000 CVD deaths in Scandinavia (though appreciably more in Japan). No equivalent terms are listed.

This is a category which will generally be ignored in the data considered below. Perhaps the modern parlance of transient ischemic attacks (TIA) will be defined as 333 in later revisions of the ISC, but at present No. 333 is a rubric of little value.

Other and ill-defined lesions (other CVD) is a repository for terms not applicable to the previous categories. It should include "apoplexy, stroke, or paralytic stroke not otherwise classified". It also includes "apoplectiform convulsions; cerebral: arteriosclerosis, arteritis, congestion, effusion, endarteritis, hemiplegia, hyperemia, monoplegia, edema, paralysis, paresis, seizure, and thrombo-angiitis obliterans"; further included are "cerebrovascular degeneration or sclerosis, intracranial congestion or effusion, sinus thrombosis of nonpyogenic origin, and thrombosis of the spinal cord". Also included here is "hypertensive encephalopathy".

Inclusion of cerebral arteriosclerosis weights this group to the aged. Hypertensive encephalopathy will have some of its members classed here, others under No. 441 (essential malignant hypertensive heart disease), and yet more under No. 445 (essential malignant hypertension). These are generally rather minor quibbles, and the basic use of No. 334 would seem to be for those instances where the clinician or the encoder is uncertain whether to list a case under 331 or 332. In certain countries (Switzerland and Israel), this class contains the vast majority of CVD deaths, which is doubtless the result of coding fashions and not a true reflection of the real situation. In general the frequency of No. 334 is inversely related to the sum of No. 331 and 332.

It might be mentioned that there is an officially-sanctioned subcoding for ISC rubric 332, in which cerebral embolism *is* separated from thrombosis, but with a third category (among others) for cerebellar thrombosis *or* embolism. Available mortality data however are not so subdivided, except in rare instances.

Clinical Definitions

We will retain the basic divisions of 330 (SAH), 331 (Cb H), 332 (Cb thr-emb), and 334 (other), and upon these build our clinical subclasses.

A. Under SAH, the major divisions will be:
a) SAH associated with aneurysm,
b) SAH associated with arteriovenous malformation (AVM),
c) SAH associated with hypertension (HT) and/or arteriosclerosis (AS),
d) SAH associated with miscellaneous diseases, such as leukemia, carcinomatosis, brain tumor, infections,
e) SAH associated with no known disease ("idiopathic" SAH).

Criteria are generally obvious to assign a case to these groups. Adequate angiography is an essential prerequisite, and of course the use of autopsy material will not be ignored. Subdivisions according to the site of aneurysm or of AVM are also appropriate.

B. Cerebral hemorrhage remains as a unit.

C. Cerebral thrombosis-embolism is divisible in several ways.
1. Pathophysiologically divisions are:
a) cerebral thrombosis
(1) "thrombosis in evolution", "ingravescent stroke", "progressive stroke". A clinical definition where deterioration continues under observation.
(2) "completed stroke", where no worsening occurs in the acute situation. This is at times used as equivalent to "thrombosis" (FISHER).

The definition of cerebral thrombosis is usually that of a relatively acute cerebral insult with no obvious external cause, manifest by focal neurologic deficits which persist for a considerable period of time, which is unassociated with evidence of intracranial bleeding by clinical and spinal fluid examination, and which may or may not receive confirmation by evidence of diseased blood vessels upon angiography. Thus "cerebral thrombosis" is in large measure a diagnosis of exclusion.

b) transient ischemic attacks (TIA) are short-lived episodes of focal neurologic dysfunction attributed to cerebrovascular disease. Duration of episodes is generally 10 min or so, and the signs and symptoms must have completely abated within a matter of 1 h (FISHER) to 24 h (MARSHALL). I would find it difficult to so class a patient with only one such episode. Pathophysiologically this group would seem to fall in the general class of cerebral thrombosis. TIA are the modern equivalents for cerebral artery spasm, one might surmise.

c) cerebral embolism refers to conditions of acute, indeed apoplectic, onset, again manifest by focal neurologic deficit, with evidence of one or several lesions. Usually included is evidence for a source of emboli, such as cardiac arhythmia, recent through-and-through myocardial infarct, rheumatic heart disease, subacute bacterial endocarditis; evidence of other emboli (petechiae of skin or retina) is also taken as confirmatory. The perhaps hypothetical fragmentation of thrombi in the carotid or vertebrobasilar trunks is generally not included in the embolic group.

d) "thorem" is a term used (FISHER) when the clinician cannot decide between *th*rombosis *or em*bolism.

2. It is also customary to divide the thrombosis-embolism group according to the anatomic site of the lesion. While formerly many pages of neurologic texts were devoted to the syndromes of individual intracranial arteries and their branches, the pendulum has swung so far as to consider the neck as the major locus of diseased blood vessels in the view of some workers. However, if we consider the trunk *and* the branches, we can appropriately divide strokes into those involving the carotid tree and the vertebrobasilar tree, the former including lesions within the anterior and middle cerebral arteries and their divisions, and the latter the vessels to the brain stem and cerebellum, and the posterior cerebral arteries. We can also consider anatomically not only the location of the vascular lesion, but also the distribution of encephalomalacia as found at autopsy.

3. Etiologic divisions are of little general value. While in a few instances the pathologic process will be states such as arteritis, the vast majority of cases are the resultant of arteriosclerotic changes in the blood vessels.

References

ad hoc Committee 9
BAKER 22

BRADSHAW 40
CARTER 53
FISHER, C. M. 104

HEYMAN 148
WHISNANT 384
World Health Organization 393

CHAPTER III

On the Validity of Mortality Data

We have seen that one important source of epidemiologic information is available in the mortality statistics published in most civilized lands, and we have considered the diagnostic subdivisions of CVD as they are classified in this regard. Some benefits and drawbacks of mortality data have already been mentioned, but the most important question to answer is how reliable are the data — to what extent can we equate death certificates with the diseases they purport to represent.

There are three ways to validate mortality data, administrative, clinical, and autopsy. Administrative review would include the check for mechanical coding errors, where the wrong diagnosis was inadvertently noted. It would also include review by a medical man to ascertain that the correct entity was chosen as the underlying cause of death. Clinical review would go beyond this point, and seek to determine from records or the treating physician the bases on which the diagnoses lay. Autopsy confirmation would seem the method *par excellence* however in this matter.

Actually, autopsy diagnosis should match completely that on the death certificate in recent years, since it is now a rather general requirement to file an amended cause-of-death statement when new information (such as autopsy) becomes available. How frequently this is effected however is conjectural.

One question is how well *should* autopsy findings correlate with the clinical. If all deaths are autopsied, then the concordance should be complete. Where only a fraction of deaths — even of hospital deaths — undergo post-mortem examination, then we may well get a fictitiously high rate of error. Obvious instances of common disease would seldom be selected for autopsy; great effort will be made to obtain a post in esoteric conditions or undiagnosed ills. With this in mind however we can look at several studies to this point.

SWARTOUT (1940) found especially good correlations between death certificates and autopsy findings for acute childhood diseases, carcinoma, tuberculosis, and blood dyscrasias among 8000 autopsies at a Los Angeles hospital; the overall rate of agreement for all diseases was 79%. For cerebrovascular disease *as a group* 90% of clinical diagnoses were correct — confirmed by autopsy, but an additional 9% were first discovered in that fashion. For subdivisions of CVD, rates were 74 and 76% correct diagnoses for cerebral hemorrhage and thrombosis-embolism, but only 16% (5/32) for "softening of the brain" (code 82c, no longer used).

POHLEN (1942) found deaths for cancer from New York hospitals were essentially correct in 88% of cases. In a later study (1943) he noted an error rate of but 14% for 19 common causes of death among 25,000 autopsies. CVD was not included.

Less sanguine were the findings of JAMES (1955) with 1900 autopsies from upstate New York: although there was only a 9% decrease in CVD deaths when autopsy data were used instead of the death certificates, this (as with most other diseases) was a net result of compensatory errors. Of the 131 CVD deaths per certificates, only 78 or 60% were retained as the underlying cause of death after autopsy. The CVD death rate in the study (7% of deaths) was well below that of upstate New York (11%), as well as that in the hospitals under study (10%), since only half the CVD hospital deaths were autopsied. I suspect most of the unautopsied were "typical" cases, of little pathologic interest, and the errors might thereby be considerably less.

More heartening was the report of ERHARDT (1959). Of some 5600 deaths due to CVD in New York, only 38 were removed and 11 added, for a net change of —0.5%, when autopsy-based revisions of diagnosis were considered. However there are no data on how many certificates should have been revised. Further only some 13% of all deaths were subject to autopsy, and this report therefore cannot speak well to the point of diagnostic accuracy.

Sox (1966) has recently discussed the validity of cardiovascular-renal death reports in San Francisco from a project which is one part of the Inter-American Mortality Investigation. For some 1800 deaths in individuals aged 15—74 between 1962 and 1964, autopsy was done in 56%, other pathologic examination in 7%, and surgery in 19%. Detailed clinical information was obtained from hospital records and/or physician interviews in 78% and from coroner or medical examiner in 22% of deaths. These patients had hospital or clinic care in their last year of life in 73% of cases and similar private physician care in 6%. The original number of deaths attributed to CVD on the standard death certificate was 279; this was raised upon review by 11.6%. Though not explicitly so stated, I have inferred that few CVD deaths were removed from the original roster because of erroneous allocation.

Thus in terms of autopsy confirmation from major population centers in this country, mortality data for CVD as a whole would appear to reflect errors of under-reporting of some 10 to 15 % (Sox, SWARTOUT), and of over-reporting of 10 (SWARTOUT) to 40% (JAMES). Subdivisions of CVD would seem far more subject to error.

In France, JUSTIN-BESANÇON (1963, 1964) reported that CVD was the under-lying cause of death in 11.7% of 1000 autopsies at a Paris hospital, and at the same time was so noted in mortality statistics from Paris in 12.1% of deaths and in the entirety of France in 12.0%. While this concordance is striking, we must recall the same individuals are not represented from both Paris sources.

MUNCK (1952) studied the correlation between clinical and pathologic causes of death in 1000 autopsies from Aarhus, Denmark, where the autopsy rate was 78% of hospital deaths. Overall, the principal disease was correctly diagnosed clinically in 80% of cases, was almost correct in 9%, was wrong in 5% and un-diagnosed in 7%. The only label used for CVD clinically was "cerebral hemorrhage" (typical of mortality data for the period). This was confirmed in but 21 (44%), and two undiagnosed instances were found at post mortem. However, of the 27 "misses", there were 18 cases of encephalomalacia and 3 subdural hematomas. Thus if we consider "cerebral hemorrhage" (as it should be in the mortality data of the 1940's and earlier) as equivalent to "CVD", then we have $21 + 18 = 39$ confirmed cases, or 81% of those so labelled clinically, and 2 cases or 5% unrecognized *in vivo*. With the subdurals, proper for coding rules, the confirmation rate is 88%.

LINELL (1964) questioned the value of mortality statistics in Sweden since only 81% of his series of fresh myocardial infarction were confirmed at autopsy. In contesting this, VON HOFSTEN (1964) pointed out that most diagnostic errors (regardless of cause) were in the elderly where multiple ills are present.

From Umeå, Sweden, OTTERLAND (1964) presented a unique study wherein the same patients were assessed from clinical diagnosis, from their death certificates as officially coded, and from autopsy data. In this hospital 98% of those who died came to autopsy! He stated that about one in three deaths in Sweden are autopsied. Of 326 cases, clinical and autopsy diagnoses were identical in 72%; there were minor differences in subclassification in 6%, and variations within the same diagnostic category in 9%. In only 13% was there a major misclassification of the primary cause of death. For the category of nervous system diseases (of which some 85% are CVD in Scandinavia), there were 38 cases so classed clinically, of which 33 were listed in the mortality statistics and 33 confirmed at autopsy, for a rate of confirmation of better than 85% on clinical basis, and 100% from the mortality data.

Accuracy of death certification in England has been studied by HEASMAN (1962) in a special project covering nearly 15,000 deaths at a number of hospitals. Although all deaths were supposed to be autopsied, this frequency actually ranged from 30 to 100%, and was strongly related to clinical uncertainty as to diagnosis and the (young) age of the patient. Only half the patients of 65 or older whose diagnosis was "fairly certain" were autopsied as opposed to some 85% when the diagnosis was "uncertain". In reconstructing his tables it would seem that there were 1839 cases in which the clinical diagnosis was some form of CVD (330 to 334) as the underlying cause of death. Of these, only 55% were autopsied. Among the 1016 autopsied cases called CVD clinically, the diagnosis was substantiated in 740 or 73%, and wrong "in fact" (disease other than CVD) in 276 or 27%. There were another 54 cases where clinical and pathologic discrepancies were noted; these were "differences of opinion or wording" and I have discarded them as not being clearly positive *or* negative. An additional 92 cases (9.1%) were first classed as CVD at post mortem. Considering that the half not autopsied would mostly be clinically "fairly certain" CVD, this rate of confirmation would appear satisfactory.

The diagnostic divisions of CVD fared less well. *Some* form of CVD was the underlying cause in 92% of SAH, 74% of hemorrhage, 62% of thrombosis, and 54% of "other" CVD. SAH was called SAH though in only 70% of instances, and in like fashion the proper labels were applied to cerebral hemorrhage in 52%, thrombosis in 48%, and "other" CVD in but 22%. His more recent elaboration of this work (1966) is essentially confirmatory of the information just cited. In the latter, HEASMAN lists the 75 hospitals of England and Wales whose deaths in part of 1959 provided the material for the study.

Therefore it would seem that CVD as a unit is correctly cited in mortality data from Europe in 73 (HEASMAN) to 100% (OTTERLAND) of cases, and missed clinically in 0 (OTTERLAND) to 9% (HEASMAN), with MUNCK's data intermediate. Thus CVD does appear to be more accurately labelled in Europe than in the United

States. Better reporting would seem a consequence of smaller countries with more uniform population groups and medical facilities, the higher proportions of deaths in hospital, and the higher rates of autopsies performed.

Further to the differentiation of cerebral hemorrhage and thrombosis, ACHESON (1966) noted that the rules governing statistical coding of death certificates artificially inflate cerebral hemorrhage, since he states the regulations call for ascribing "cerebrovascular accident" or "stroke" to ISC rubric 331. This is incorrect (see prior chapter), but may well be the rule under which he and FLOREY (1967) had to work; FLOREY's paper is basically "administrative review". KRUEGER (1967) did not allocate the non-specific entities to 331 in his survey of CVD deaths in Memphis. Even in Europe though the error rate for the subdivisions of CVD was in the order of 30 to 80% (HEASMAN).

Differences in diagnostic fashion or acumen would not appear a likely cause of the variations between either side of the Atlantic. From a review of the same small sample of patient charts, REID (1964) indicated good uniformity among physicians of Great Britain, the United States, and Norway. For example, 19, 20, and 22% of deaths were attributed to CVD in the respective countries. Again however the CVD subdivisions were much more discrepant, ranging from 9 to 13% for hemorrhage, 4 to 9% for thrombosis, and 0.3 to 4.4% for "other" CVD, with no consistent national preferences.

A complex mathematical factor analysis by GRIFFITH (1961) purports to speak to the point of diagnostic accuracy in various diseases, based upon English male mortality rates for 22 common diseases. After removing the effects of age and socioeconomic status, about half the residual variance for CVD, common cancers, and renal disease fell into the components he equates with diagnostic error. DIAMOND (1962) and NEWELL (1962) discussed the effects of misclassification in epidemiology. Other papers dealing with autopsy validation but without specific reference to stroke include those of HAMTOFT (1961), WAALER (1958), and ZSCHOCH (1959, 1964). We shall consider JABLON's work (1966) in the chapter (VIII) dealing with race in CVD.

Realizing that autopsy material is likely to be biased, MORIYAMA (1958) sought a different method to validate mortality statistics. He asked the certifying physician to review the clinical data underlying some 2000 death certificates in Pennsylvania, and this material together with the original death certificates were then reviewed by his group for diagnostic adequacy and accuracy. In the context of all available data, in 85% of the 254 CVD deaths this was deemed the most probable diagnosis, in 9% another diagnosis was equally probable, and in 2% an alternative was preferred. MORIYAMA (1966) extended this study upon some 1400 cardiovascular deaths obtained from a two-month national sample of deaths in 1960. Questionnaires were sent to the certifying physician and all material was review by internists. Of the 449 CVD deaths, 14% were considered well established, 41% reasonable with incomplete evidence, and 17% reasonable with no diagnostic evidence (total 72%); in 15% the evidence was insufficient to support any diagnosis, and for 12% there was no useful response to the survey. The number of CVD cited is an increase of 5% over the original death certificates, a result of the group's reallocation after review. We should remember though that these last studies comprise diagnostic "concensus" rather than diagnostic "proof". More importantly

though all the United States data cited come largely from the major population
centers of presumably advanced medical care. For example, the number of
physicians per capita in New York in 1962 was 145% of the national mean;
similar figures for California were 126, for Massachusetts 139, and for Pennsylvania
109% of the mean. Lastly, the information refers predominantly to the white
citizens. As will be seen in Chapter VIII, reliability in the Negro is a far different
question.

Are then mortality data sufficiently accurate for use in stroke? I think the
answer is "yes" — for CVD as a whole and in the lands we considered above. One
statistician has said that characteristics of a group should be definable if the group
is some 70% "pure" (accurately classed). The "impurities" will be heterogeneous
and will serve but to dilute the features present in the true class. Any major
("important") variable of CVD should then show through these impurities with
the assessment of these mortality data. For the subdivisions of CVD though, error
rates of 30 to 80% really preclude any confidence in the material.

References

ACHESON 5	JAMES 162	OTTERLAND 276
DIAMOND 78, 79	JUSTIN-BESANÇON 166, 167	POHLEN 295, 296
ERHARDT 96	KNOX 180	REID 301
FLOREY 112	KRUEGER 185	SOX 334
GRIFFITH 130	LINELL 202	SWARTOUT 354
HAMTOFT 142	MORIYAMA 258, 259	VON HOFSTEN 375
HEASMAN 146 (1), (2)	MUNCK 263	WAALER 376
JABLON 161	NEWELL 268	ZSCHOCH 410, 411

CHAPTER IV

General Features of Cerebral Vascular Disease

To begin the epidemiology of CVD, we shall in this chapter look at its general distribution by country and age. We will consider "stroke" as one entity, and later note wherein the parts differ from the whole. The materials used are chiefly mortality statistics and population surveys. Our prime question here then is how common in general is CVD — and in whom.

In this and the succeeding chapters the information will be set forth in graphs and but few tables. The basic data underlying both are presented in the Appendix tables, in detail more than adequate for most purposes. All data, whether from official national publications or from individual papers, have been checked and usually recast; appropriate statistical tests have been applied in almost all instances.

Mortality Data. A valuable contribution to the epidemiology of neurologic disease is the paper of GOLDBERG (1962), who presented graphs comparing international mortality rates for a number of disorders. All rates were from the 1951—58 period and were age-standardized to the United States population; the tabular data underlying GOLDBERG's figure for CVD mortality rates were published by STALLONES (1965). Of the 33 countries included, I chose the 18 which appeared to me most likely to have adequate medical and reporting standards. Further I deliberately omitted the U. S. Negro and Japanese rates, not only here but in the entirely of this and the following chapters. They are separately covered in the Chapter VIII on race.

In Table IV—1 are the age-adjusted average annual mortality rates for CVD deaths among these 18 countries, expressed as cases per 100,000 population. The weighted mean for all 18 was 99.46, or 1 death from CVD each year for every

Table IV—1. *Age-adjusted average annual mortality rates, deaths per 100,000 population, 1951—1958**

A. All cerebrovascular disease (330—334)

Country	rate	Country	rate	Country	rate
Norway	97.9	Scotland	148.1	Italy	125.1
Sweden	103.8	Ireland	98.2	Canada	96.6
Denmark	99.5	France	98.5	USA (white)	94.8
Finland	152.5	Netherlands	96.7	Australia	118.0
Iceland	105.7	Belgium	48.3	New Zealand	101.5
England-Wales	116.2	Switzerland	109.1	U.So.Africa (white)	101.2

weighted mean = 99.46

* study of GOLDBERG, whose data were cited by STALLONES.

1000 people. Most of the countries were rather close to this figure, though Finland (153) and Scotland (148) were high and Belgium (48) quite low; this last is rather surprising, since the rates in contiguous countries were near the mean rate. All three discrepant rates though are based on rather small populations and this could be chance variation.

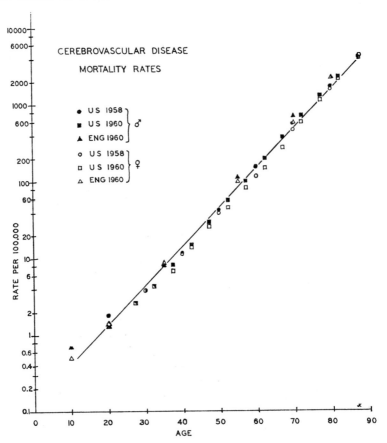

Fig. IV−1. Age and sex specific annual mortality rates for CVD deaths in cases per 100,000 population, for whites in the United States (1958, 1960), and for England and Wales (1960), plotted against age on a logarithmic scale for the rates. Data are in Appendix Table IV−a−1, from BERKSON (1965), DU BOULAY (1965), and WYLIE [1961, 1962 (1)]

We know quite well that stroke is a disease of the elderly, but the extent of its shift to the senium may not be fully appreciated. As we shall see, about $^3/_4$ of all CVD deaths are reported in individuals age 70 or older.

There are two ways to attain comparability of mortality (or prevalence) rates in different lands; the common one is that already cited, adjusting for age to a standard population. Another way though — and the method underlying age-standardization — is to present the age-specific rates. A simple means for presentation is to plot the age-specific rates against age on a graph, and this was done for this work. When the rates were plotted on a logarithmic scale, it was apparent that the CVD curves were linear, and, as we shall see, were all generally the *same* curve. Fig. IV–1 is the graph for age-specific annual mortality rates for CVD in the United States and England, for each sex; data for this figure are in Appendix Table IV–a–1. Two features stand out to me: first, the same line looks like the best fit for each country; second, differences between sexes are minimal compared

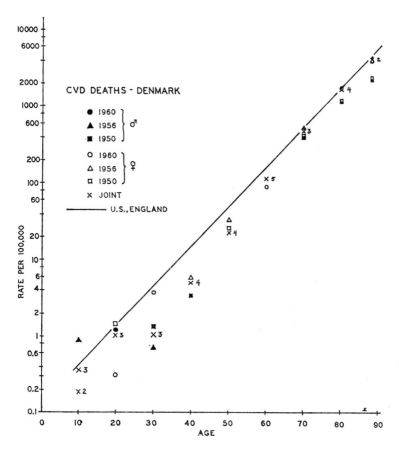

Fig. IV–2. Age and sex specific annual mortality rates for CVD deaths in cases per 100,000 population in Denmark 1950, 1956, 1960. Solid line represents US-England. Date are presented in Appendix Tables IV–a–2, 5, 6, 7

with the differences between any two consecutive age groups. Also, it made no difference whether ages were divided in 5-year or 10-year periods, or even 20-year periods. So impressive (to me) was this curve that I used it as the standard in all the other CVD data based on population rates.

In Fig. IV–2, age-specific CVD death rates are plotted for Denmark for the years 1950, 1956, and 1960. Generally speaking the rates are lower than our standard in the younger ages where cases are few, and tend to reach the "standard" line in the older ages, where cases are much more numerous. A logarithmic scale exaggerates differences at the lower end and minimizes them at the upper. Data

2*

for this figure are in Appendix Tables IV—a—2, 5, 6, 7, and were obtained from the sources cited in the references (det Statistiske Department; Sundhedsstyrelsen).

As an aside, the years chosen for Scandinavian studies here were those previously used in an evaluation of multiple sclerosis, for which I had amassed a considerable amount of demographic information (KURTZKE, 1965—67). I had planned

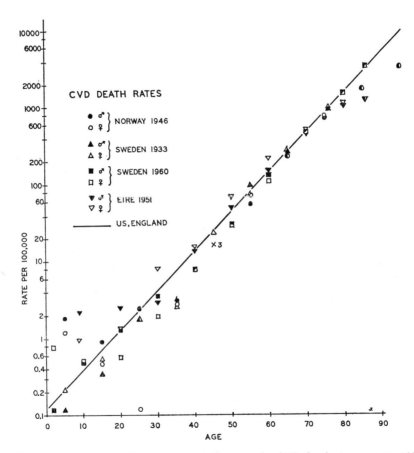

Fig. IV—3. Age and sex specific annual mortality rates for CVD deaths in cases per 100,000 population in Norway (1946), Sweden (1933, 1960), and Ireland (1951). Solid line represents US-England. Data are presented in Appendix Tables IV—a—8 thru-11

to evaluate also data from each Scandinavian country for 1960, but did not do so for Norway since the results were almost monotonously the same.

Similar age-specific mortality rates for CVD deaths are presented in Fig. IV—3. I think one can see what I mean about similar results. Quite interesting are the findings for Sweden: rates in 1933 are the same as those almost 30 years later. Also, the US-England line still looks like the best fit. A drift away from the line at the uppermost ages — even though large in absolute cases and rates — must be viewed with caution; cases are more than adequate in number, but the *population* at this end is so small that it provides unstable rates, a situation quite unique.

The data for Fig. IV—3 are in Appendix Tables IV—a—8 through 11, and were obtained from standard sources as cited (Statistisk Sentralbyrå for Norway, Statistika Centralbyrån for Sweden, Central Statistical Office for Eire).

Similar results were apparent for CVD deaths in Italy in 1953—55 and 1959—61 (BIANCONE, 1964), but have not been entabled. The most recent study available

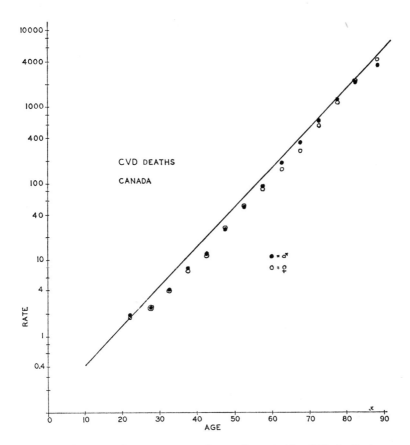

Fig. IV—4. Age and sex specific average annual mortality rates for CVD deaths in cases per 100,000 population in Canada (1960—1964). Solid line represents US-England. Data are in Appendix Table IV—a—12, from P. C. GORDON (1966)

was however added. Plotting the CVD mortality rates for Canada, as provided by P. C. GORDON (1966), gives us still a quite good agreement with our US-England "standard" (Fig. IV—4).

A somewhat unique view of mortality statistics is that provided by Sox (1966) as a part of an inter-American cooperative study on validation of mortality data. An appropriate sample of all deaths occurring in 1962—64 in San Francisco, California, among those age 15 to 74 were reviewed, with retrieval of the medical information as well as the death certificate. Therefore his diagnoses for CVD deaths are as accurate as possible without 100% autopsy rates. Naturally the

CVD numbers are small, being in fact 0 to 6 for the first three age groups in either sex (Appendix Table IV—a—13). I think this study provides an excellent validation for our use of the US-England curve for age-specific CVD mortality rates. It may be worth reiterating that there seems to be essential equality between the sexes from these age-specific rates (Fig. IV—5).

In addition to categorizing CVD deaths as a proportion of the population, in whole or by age-group, we can also see what proportion of *deaths* are attributed

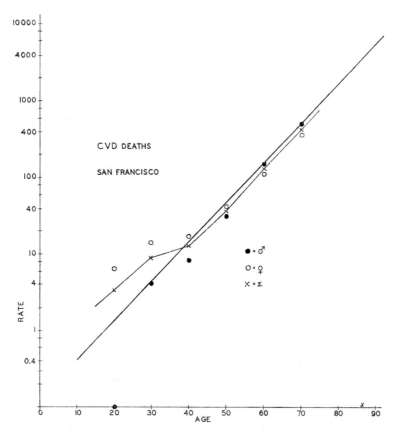

Fig. IV—5. Age and sex specific average annual mortality rates for CVD deaths in cases per 100,000 population between age 15 and 74 in San Francisco, California (1962—1964). Heavy solid line represents US-England. Light line connects the age-specific rates for both sexes combined. Data are in Appendix Table IV−a−13, from Sox (1966)

to CVD. This ratio is not a good one for general epidemiologic use since it is obvious that many factors in which we have no immediate interest go into making up the denominator. It has its clinical analog in classification of autopsies by the proportions found due to various entities. In Appendix Table IV—a—3, the percentages of CVD deaths to total deaths in Denmark in 1950 are listed by age and sex. CVD are about 0.5% under age 15, 1 to 2% age 15 to 44, 4% at age 45 to 54, and between 7 and 11% in the older groups. The relative frequency of CVD as a cause of death in the elderly is summarized in Table IV−2. The CVD rate at present would seem to be the order of 15% of deaths in those age 60 or 65 and older, taking the Danish and Swedish frequencies. The former has risen appreciably over the previous ten years, which again shows the unsatisfactory nature of this means of comparison, since the age-specific mortality rates were very similar.

Table IV−2. *Relative frequency of deaths due to cerebrovascular disease in the elderly*

Country and year	age	sex	all deaths (A)	CVD deaths (B)	Percentage (B)/(A)
Ireland 1951	60 ≤	M	15,788	1,152	7.3
		F	14,595	1,397	9.6
		Σ	30,383	2,549	8.4
Norway 1946	60 ≤	M	8,638	1,085	12.6
		F	10,137	1,431	14.1
		Σ	18,775	2,516	13.4
Denmark 1950	65 ≤	M	11,935	1,144	9.6
		F	12,947	1,427	11.0
		Σ	24,882	2,571	10.3
Denmark 1960	65 ≤	M	15,135	2,117	14.0
		F	14,990	2,590	17.3
		Σ	30,125	4,707	15.6
Sweden av. 1956—1960	65 ≤	M	25,413	3,805	15.0
		F	25,963	4,978	19.2
		Σ	51,376	8,783	17.1

Incidence Data. The frequency of the occurence of CVD is poorly determined by the frequency of deaths so attributed. There have been several population surveys though which give us direct information on the incidence of strokes.

In EISENBERG's study (1964) of Middlesex, Connecticut, he found that 191 previously healthy adults suffered a stroke in 1957—58. Their ages at ictus for each sex are shown in Fig. IV−6, as the percentage frequencies of total CVD; data are in Appendix Table IV−a−14. These frequencies are superimposed on the similar curve for CVD deaths in Denmark in 1950. It would appear that there is not much difference between the two, and this is indeed generally true: as percentages of all CVD, distributions of age at ictus and at death will be quite similar. However, when we return to our population base, the picture changes.

A similar population study for stroke was carried out in 1957 in Rochester, Minnesota by KURLAND (1967). Adding his series to EISENBERG's on a weighted basis (Appendix Table IV−a−15), we can delineate an age-specific incidence rate curve for CVD in the United States, based on 255 patients. This curve with its 95% confidence limits is drawn in Fig. IV−7. We can see that the incidence or attack rates between age 35 and 74 are considerably (and significantly) higher than our "standard" death rates; indeed they are about twice as great. This would *suggest* that the case-fatality rate for stroke might be in the order of 50% of all CVD below age 75, and that case-fatality rates might rise with age, since the incidence curve meets the mortality curve at the 85-and-over age.

There have been several other population surveys from which age-specific incidence rates for CVD have been or could be calculated.

In an intensive survey of Carlisle, England, BREWIS (1966) has documented the population characteristics of a large number of neurologic diseases, among which of course is CVD. There were 694 cases in the 1955—61 period. PARRISH (1966)

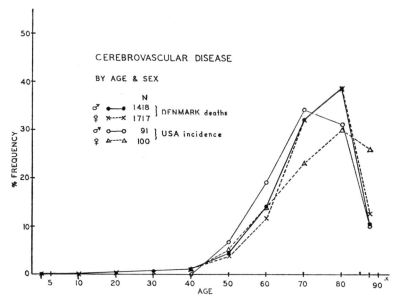

Fig. IV–6. Percentage frequency distribution of CVD cases by age and sex, from Connecticut incidence (1957—1958) and Danish mortality (1950) series. Data for Middlesex, Connecticut are in Appendix Table IV–a–14, from EISENBERG (1964), and for Denmark in Table IV–a–2

conducted a survey for stroke in three mid-Missouri counties in 1963—64, with 195 cases discovered. An intensive morbidity survey throughout England and Wales was accomplished in 1955—56; reports from 106 general practices provided almost 1,900 CVD cases (LOGAN, 1958; Research Committee of the Council of the College of General Practitioners, 1962). The age-specific annual incidence rates from these works are drawn in Fig. IV—8, and the data are in Appendix Tables IV—a—17 and 19. In the major portion of the distribution, the two population surveys of Carlisle and Missouri are quite similar to the Middlesex-Rochester series. In the lowest ages of course we have in all studies the most uncertain rates. The Carlisle attack rate tapers off with age, and indeed eventually falls below the US-England CVD death line, while the Missouri series stays within the confidence limits for the Middlesex-Rochester rates. The decline in Carlisle may well be caused by the fact that for stroke (unlike other entities studied), BREWIS had to rely on hospital data for almost all her cases. It is likely that hospitalization was less routine for the oldest patients with stroke.

The rates reported from the British general practices are considerably the highest from any source. Numbers too are appreciable. Because the cases were grouped differently from those of the other incidence studies, I did not test the differences for statistical significance. If we assume these rates are "truly" higher,

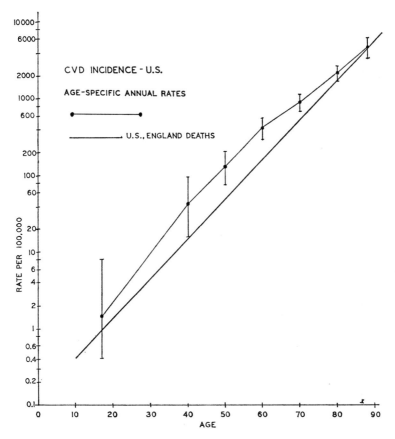

Fig. IV–7. Age specific annual incidence rates for CVD in cases per 100,000 population, with 95% confidence limits on the rates, from weighted averages for cases from population surveys of Middlesex, Connecticut (1957—1958), and Rochester, Minnesota (1957). Heavy solid line represents US-England mortality rates. Data are in Appendix Tables IV–a–15, from EISEN-BERG (1964) and KURLAND (1967) respectively

a facile explanation is hard to come by since none of our other material suggests any appreciable difference between US and English strokes. It is of some interest that this rate and the Carlisle rate run close to the upper and lower confidence limits respectively from the Middlesex-Rochester stroke rates. I am inclined to pass off as within the bounds of chance the apparent excess from LOGAN's study.

Validation for portions of the age-specific US incidence rates is present too in other more restricted studies. BERKSON (1965) cited surveys among employees in

Delaware and Chicago. KANNEL's Framingham study (1965) and two age-limited New York assessments by LADD (1962) also give us some information. The age-specific rates in each instance fall well within the range of those from Rochester-Middlesex (Appendix Table IV—a—16).

There is yet another community survey in which all the CVD cases in Goulburn, Australia were recorded (and examined) by WALLACE (1967). Unfortunately

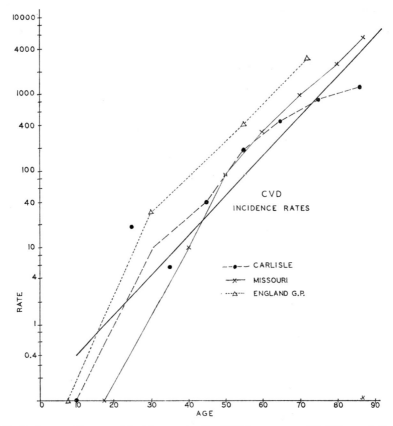

Fig. IV—8. Age specific annual incidence rates for CVD in cases per 100,000 population from several other population surveys: Carlisle, England (1955—1961), three mid-Missouri counties (1963—1964), and 106 general practices in England and Wales (1955—1956). Heavy solid line represents US-England mortality rates. Data are in Appendix Table IV—a—17 for Carlisle (BREWIS, 1966) and Missouri (PARRISH, 1966), and in IV—a—19 for the general practices (LOGAN, 1958)

population ages were not provided, so the cases are distributed as percentages of the total CVD by age (Fig. IV—9, data in Appendix Table IV—a—18).

DALSGAARD-NIELSEN (1955) described the characteristics of 1,000 CVD cases from 1940 to 1953 in Frederiksberg, Denmark. Though this was a hospital series, medical practice in the area was such that one might have expected most strokes to appear on his rolls. In point of fact however, age-specific annual incidence rates calculated from this material are quite uniformly about half those from the popu-

lation surveys we have considered, and an even smaller proportion in the oldest
ages (Appendix Table IV—a—20). Other hospital series cannot be used to speak
to the point of incidence of the disease, but they do provide us with some information on the sex ratios in CVD.

Sex Ratios in CVD. Much has been made of a purported lower frequency of
strokes in young women and their accelerated acquisition of this disorder with age.
This has even been used as a rationale for steroid therapy in strokes. We have
already seen, however, from both the incidence and the mortality works considered,
that any sex difference would seem minimal at best. More to the point though

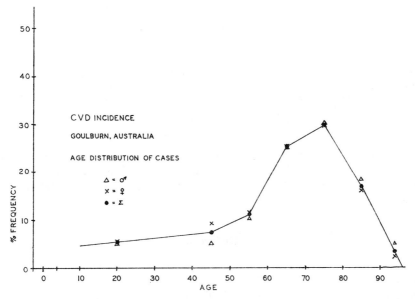

Fig. IV—9. Percentage frequency distribution by age and sex for CVD cases from incidence
study in Goulburn, Australia (1962—1964). Data are in Appendix Table IV—a—18, from
WALLACE (1967)

would be direct assessment. In Appendix Table IV—a—21 are listed sex ratios of
CVD from some 15 mortality studies. Male/female ratios are derived both from the
numbers of cases and from the sex-specific mortality rates. Median ages are listed.
For CVD deaths in all ages the ratios from the rates (which are the more valid)
range from 0.78 to 1.03. For series limited to younger strokes the ratios are 1.04
to 1.28. In the next part of the table we see ratios from eight large hospital series
and six population surveys. Hospital series ratios based on cases range from 0.69
to 1.25 (one hospital's ratio was 1.75 while its ratio for all admissions was 1.63).
In two instances ratios based on population rates were 1.16 (median age 74) and
0.88 (age 70). The population survey M/F ratios based on cases ranged from
0.72 to 1.06, and on rates from 0.87 to 1.37, this last instance with only 64 cases.
In neither of these sources was there any obvious relation of the ratios to age.

Since however there seemed to be a suggestion of a decreased female frequency
in the young in the mortality data, this required further definition, and the

Table IV–3. *Male/Female Ratios from age-specific mortality rates for all CVD*

Age	Source										Un-weighted Average
	(1)	(2)	(3)	(4)	(5)	(6)	(7)	(8)	(9)	(10)	
25—34*	1.03	—	—	—	—	0.37	1.36	0.70	0.31	1.85	0.94
35—44*	1.05	—	—	—	—	0.88	0.68	1.02	0.67	1.00	0.88
45—54	1.19	0.95	1.00	0.86	0.64	0.73	0.96	0.74	1.01	1.04	0.91
55—64	1.34	1.15	1.14	1.06	0.73	0.68	1.05	1.02	1.25	1.19	1.06
65—74	1.27	1.13	1.17	1.07	0.85	0.88	0.90	0.96	1.08	0.98	1.03
75—84	1.10	1.08	1.09	0.99	0.94	0.90	0.95	0.93	0.90	0.94	0.98
85 ≤	0.87	—	—	—	0.94	0.99	0.97	1.13	0.97	1.04	0.99
Total	0.94	—	—	—	0.94	0.79	0.84	0.86	0.86	0.84	0.87

* rates unstable due to small numbers of cases

(1) US white 1958 (WYLIE, 1961)
(2) US white 1949 (WYLIE, 1962)
(3) England-Wales 1958 (WYLIE, 1962)
(4) England-Wales 1949 (WYLIE, 1962)
(5) Eire 1946—1955 (ACHESON, 1960)

(6) Eire 1951
(7) Denmark 1950
(8) Denmark 1956
(9) Denmark 1960
(10) Sweden 1960

obvious method was to calculate the sex ratios for age specific CVD death rates. The results are in Table IV–3. To me, this indicates there is no real difference between the sexes for CVD deaths, and, with the variability in hospital and population series, no real difference either for CVD cases.

References

Mortality data
ACHESON, R. M. 2, 6
BERKSON 30
BIANCONE 31
BORHANI 36, 37
BURGESS 49
Central Statistics Office 55
CRAWFORD 64
DU BOULAY 87
FUMAGALLI 116
General Register Office 118
GOLDBERG 125
GORDON, P. C. 128
Kungl. Medicinalstyrelsen 186
KURTZKE 189—194
SOX 334
STAMLER 335
STALLONES 336

Statistisk Sentralbyrå 338—340
Statistiska Centralbyrån 341—346
det Statistiske Departement 347
Sundhedsstyrelsen 349
U. S. Bureau of the Census 370—373
WALKER 378
WYLIE 396, 397

Hospital series
ADAMS 7
CARROLL, D. 51
DALAL 69
DALSGAARD 70
FELGER 101
MARSHALL 222

NAIK 265
ZIELKE 409

Populations surveys
BERKSON 30
BORHANI 38
BREWIS 41
CHAPMAN 56
DAWBER 73
EISENBERG 93
ERICSON 97
KANNEL 169, 170
KURLAND 188
LADD 195
LOGAN 207
PARRISH 283
Research Committee 303
WALLACE 379

CHAPTER V

The Geographic Distribution of CVD

We have seen that the age-adjusted mortality rates for CVD are quite similar among 18 countries whose medical and reporting standards appear reliable. We have also shown the very striking similarities for age-specific annual mortality rates within the United States, England and Wales, Eire, Norway, Sweden, and Denmark. This would indicate that, for the lands in question, the international distribution of CVD would appear quite uniform. Let us now investigate the geographic distribution *within* these lands.

The method used to ascertain the local geographic distribution has been outlined in the first chapter, and is described in more detail elsewhere (KURTZKE, 1965—67) in connection with work on the distribution of multiple sclerosis; this work in fact determined the times of inquiry for CVD in several of these lands. In brief, we allocate the death cases by county of residence, determine the mortality rate for each county and for the entire land, and calculate the χ-square statistic for the distribution by county based on the null hypothesis of homogeneity. Mortality rates for the counties are also expressed as their percentages of the national mean mortality rate. When there is a statistically significant deviation from homogeneity, the deviations are large, *and* the high-rate areas tend to form a cluster or focus, then the association of the disease with environmental factor(s) would seem highly probable. When there is no significant deviation, *or* when (even if there is), the truly high-rate areas are few and far between, then it would appear that environmental factor(s) play no important rôle in the acquisition or manifestation of our disease. The level of statistical significance I use here to reject homogeneity is 1% (P < 0.01). By "large deviations" I have been using the criterion that several areas at least must be well beyond 25% of the national mean rate (outside 75 to 125% of the mean). In the evaluation of CVD distribution I have paid more attention to the degree and location of the deviations than to the level of statistical significance, because of the very large numbers of cases we have to deal with. The statistical texts used have been referred to in Chapter I.

In evaluating local distributions, the use of the total population of each area is satisfactory for most disorders. However the concentration of CVD in the senium makes this a rather hazardous assumption. It was impossible to obtain CVD deaths stratified by age and county, with one limited exception. A breakdown of CVD deaths in Denmark by age, sex, and rural-provincial-capital areas did not suggest marked discrepancies (Appendix Table V—a—16). However, it was soon discovered that total population denominators were in fact very misleading, and what I have used as denominator in the geographic distributions is the population age 60 and over in each area of each country. Special demographic data were kindly provided me by Adin (1964) of Sweden, Alsing (1964, 1966) and Laurssen (1963) of Denmark, and Sodeland (1964) of Norway. Other sources are cited in the references.

Sweden. In Table V–1 is a summary of the geographic distribution of CVD deaths by county for population age 60 and over, for the years 1933 and 1960. The names of the counties as well as the basic data are found in Appendix Tables V–a–5 through 9; included are geographic distributions of medical facilities (physicians and hospitals) in 1933, which were used in correlating these factors with CVD distributions.

The findings are presented (Table V–1) as percentages of the national mean rate that the mortality rate for the individual county represents. All values above 100% are of course above the national mean. Also noted is the level of statistical significance (5% level) for each area vs. the mean. The total χ-square value is cited at the bottom as 97 for 1933 (with some 1,500 CVD cases) and 219 for 1960 (with some 10,000 cases), both obviously "significant".

The CVD distributions for 1933 are drawn in Fig. V–1 as percentile ranges of the national mean rate. Both cases and populations are from "urban" areas only. All open counties are below the national mean, and the legend describes the ranges for those above the mean. We can see several features. First, most of the land area of Sweden is occupied by "high-frequency" CVD counties. Second, the highest areas are at either end of the country. With this and with so many regions "high" it seems inappropriate to consider clustering of cases as a feature here. The range of CVD rates among the counties of Sweden is from 69% to 189% of the mean. Although cases are certainly not randomly scattered and the degree of variation is large, there does not appear to be much of a pattern to the distribution.

Table V–1. *Sweden — Distribution of CVD deaths (pop. 60 ≤) by county, 1933 vs. 1960, percentages of mean mortality rate*

Area	1933	1960
1	83	77
1a	116	100
2	78	69
3	130–**	108
4	118*	97
5	119	101
6	126	96
7	86	106
8	139	107
9	153**	94
10	131	94
11	89	92
12	80	111*
13	69	89
14	116	95
15	113	120**
16	122	126**
17	122	119**
18	93	96
19	107	103
20	145**	100
21	176**	130**
22	135	114*
23	189**	111*
24	142*	123**
Total	100	100
χ^2	97.34	218.59

** = significantly high ($\chi_a^2 >$ 4.0)

* = high of dubious significance (χ_a^2 2.0—4.0)

The 1960 distribution of CVD deaths in Sweden looks quite different (Table V–1). The range is now much less, being from 69 to 130% of the mean, and only two widely separated areas barely surpass our arbitrary cut-off of 125% as being "really" high: No. 16 at 126%, and No. 21 at 130%. Despite this, the χ-square value is much larger than in the earlier study, which illustrates the point made

previously about high values with small differences when numbers are large;
there were seven times as many stroke deaths in the 1960 study.

This distribution is drawn in Fig. V—2 in precisely the same fashion as the
previous figure. Included here are the Norwegian findings which will be covered
next. Immediately obvious is the much more homogeneous nature of Swedish
stroke deaths in 1960. Our high southern "focus" of 1933 is now below the mean.
In formal testing, the correlation coefficient between 1933 and 1960 strokes was

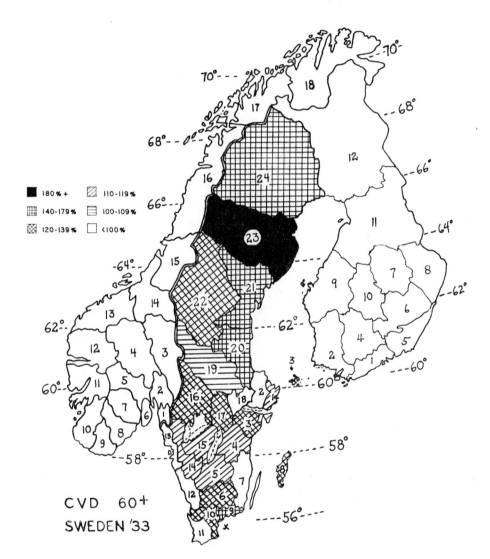

Fig. V—1. Distribution of urban CVD deaths by county in Sweden (1933) against urban
population age 60 and over, in percentile ranges of the national mean mortality rate. Data
are summarized in Table V—1 and detailed in Appendix Table V—a—5. The map is that of
Scandinavia by counties, with Norway (No. 1—18) on the left, Sweden (No. 1—24) in the
middle, and Finland (No. 1—12) on the right

+ 0.46 (0.05 > P > 0.01). As to the location of even these modestly high areas, those which exceed 110% of the mean tend to collect in two regions, one south (No. 12, 15, 16, 17), and one north (No. 21 to 24). But the northern "focus" comprises half the country. The "really" high areas (No. 16 and 21) are rather distant.

In order to illustrate how discrepant are the findings when we use the total population as the base, these CVD rates for 1960 are drawn in Fig. V–3 on a separate map of Sweden in precisely the same fashion as previous. The data for these are in Appendix Table V–a–6. The dissimilarities are obvious, I believe.

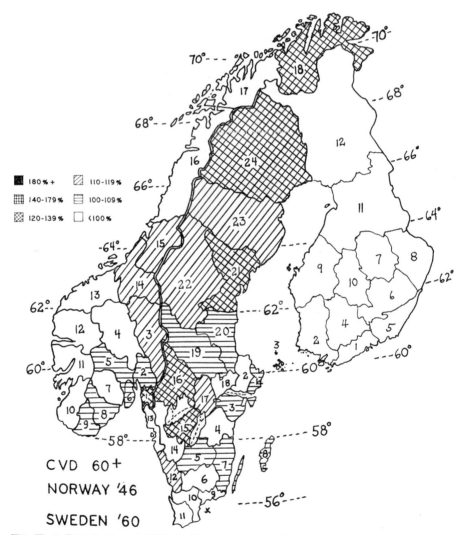

Fig. V–2. Distribution of CVD deaths by county in Sweden (1960) and Norway (1946) against populations age 60 and over, expressed in percentile ranges of the respective national mean mortality rates. Summary of data for Sweden (center) is in Table V–1 and for Norway (left) in Table V–2. Detailed data are in Appendix Tables V–a–7 and 2

To return then, because of the low degree of variation in 1960 and the relative scatter of high areas, I am forced to conclude that there is no good evidence for intrinsic geographic clustering of CVD deaths in Sweden. The relationship of the 1933 distribution to those of medical facilities will be considered later.

Norway. The CVD deaths in 1946 were allocated by county of residence. Their assessment with the total population as base is in Appendix Table V–a–1, and

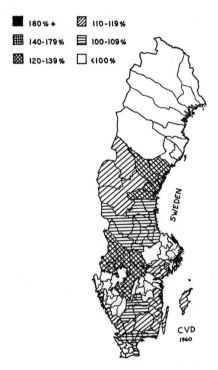

■ 180%+   ▨ 110-119%
▦ 140-179%   ▤ 100-109%
▨ 120-139%   ☐ ‹100%

Fig. V–3. Distribution of the same CVD deaths by county in Sweden (1960) as in Fig. V–2, with however the total population used as the base. Area boundaries on the map should be ignored; they delineate domsagor (smaller administrative units). Data are in the Appendix Table V–a–6

Table V–2. *Norway — Distribution of CVD deaths 1946 by county comparison of total population vs. $60 \leq$ pop. as base*

Area	Total	$60 \leq$
	% mean mortality rate	
1	123**	123**
2	99	102
3	114*	114*
4	85—	84
5	111	102
6	112	107
7	95	86
8	131**	103
9	115	103
10	72	77
11	80	81
12	118*	99
13	105	99
14	110	111
15	120—*	120—*
16	89	98
17	83	99
18	90	136**
Total	100	100
χ^2	64.47	45.64

** = significantly high ($\chi_a^2 >$ 4.0)
* = high of dubious significance (χ_a^2 2.0—4.0)

with that age 60 and over as base in V–a–2. A summary of both these distributions is provided in Table V–2. Differences are apparent, especially for the northern counties.

Here too in the formal sense there is a "significant" difference from homogeneity, with the total χ-square value of 46 for population of 60 and over (P = 0.01 at 33.4). However, the range is only from 77 to 136% of the mean, and only one area (No. 18 at 136%) reaches our criterion of outside of 25% of the mean. Further, the two highest counties (No. 1, 18) are at opposite ends of the country.

Therefore, with the small degree of variation and the absence of clustering, I would interpret this distribution as indicating that there is no biologically significant concentration of CVD deaths in Norway.

Denmark. For 1950 the only available data for the geographic distribution of CVD was that of deaths due to all neurologic diseases (other than polio, meningococcal meningitis, encephalitis, brain tumors, and trauma). Of these, 85% were CVD deaths, and this rate was the same in rural and provincial areas, in the capital, and in hospital deaths. The small numbers of non-stroke deaths therefore should not bias appreciably our findings. All Danish basic data are in Appendix Tables V—a—10 thru 16.

Distribution of the "CVD" deaths (= neurologic deaths) in 1950 among the

Table V–3. *Denmark — Comparison of distributions by county of CVD deaths, expressed as percentages of mean mortality rate for cases per 100,000 population age 60 ≤, 1950—1960*

Area	1950	1960
1	89	81
2	72	107
3	109	106
4	81	86
5	104	108
6	77	107
7	132**	112
8	107	111
9	82	99
10	106	131**
11	118**	118**
12	118*	130**
13	111*	98
14	100	91
15	113*	102
16	99	115**
17	139**	102
18	105	105
19	107	108
20	105	112*
21	109	88
22	121*	110—
23	96	114
Total	100	100
χ^2	73.33	134.41

** = significantly high ($\chi_a^2 >$ 4.0)

 * = high of dubious significance (χ_a^2 2.0—4.0)

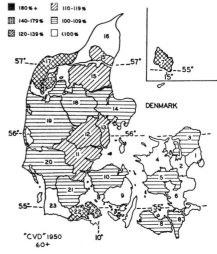

Fig. V–4. Distribution of "CVD" deaths by county in Denmark (1950) against population age 60 and over, in percentiles of the national mean mortality rate. Data are summarized in Table V–3 and detailed in Appendix Table V–a–11

23 counties of Denmark is summarized in Table V–3, together with that for (true) CVD in 1960; both are against the population age 60 and over. Again the *range* is quite small, being 72 to 139% of the mean with these 3700 cases. Only two counties (No. 7 at 131%, and No. 17 at 139%) exceed our criterion. In Fig. V–4 these findings are drawn as previous in percentiles of the national mean rate. I doubt if it would be possible to scatter more widely the three highest counties (No. 7, 17, 22).

The distribution can also be shown in terms of the level of statistical significance of the differences between individual areas and the national mean. This is a particularly good method when our rates are based on small numbers, and particularly bad with massive numbers. Here, as we can see in Fig. V–5, three scattered areas (No. 7, 11, 17) are "significantly" high and four others (No. 12, 13, 15, 22) are "high of dubious significance".

Regardless of how we assess these data, the conclusion must be negative in reference to clustering of "CVD" cases in Denmark in 1950.

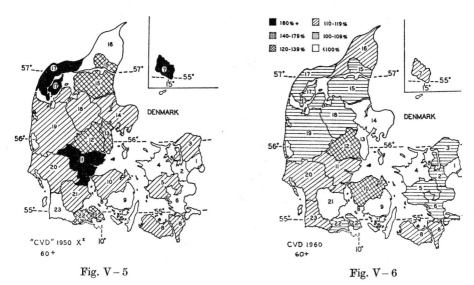

Fig. V – 5   Fig. V – 6

Fig. V–5. Distribution of "CVD" deaths by county in Denmark (1950) against population age 60 and over, in "approximate χ-square" ranges. Solid areas are "significantly" high ($\chi_a^2 > 4.0$), cross hatched are "high of dubious significance" (χ_a^2 2.0—4.0), diagonal lined areas are "insignificantly" above the mean ($\chi_a^2 < 2.0$), and open areas are below the national mean mortality rate. Data are in Appendix Table V–a–11

Fig. V–6. Distribution of CVD deaths by county in Denmark (1960), against population age 60 and over, in percentiles of the national mean mortality rate. Data are summarized in Table V–3 and detailed in Appendix Table V–a–15

The findings for 5300 stroke deaths in 1960 are as listed in Table V–3. The range now is somewhat smaller than it was in 1950, being but 81 to 131% of the mean. Two areas, this time No. 10 (131%) and No. 12 (130%), are the only ones beyond our criterion. Fig. V–6 indicates the distributions in the same percentiles of the national mean. The differences between 1950 and 1960 are quite marked I believe. In like manner we can compare the maps based on levels of significance for high-rate areas (Fig. V–7). The "significantly high" areas are now four in number (No. 10, 11, 12, 16) and only No. 11 is common to both decades. In formal testing there is no significant association between the 1950 and 1960 distributions (r = + 0.28).

Each period looked markedly different from those drawn here when total population was used as the base (see appendix tables).

It was possible also to determine the geographic distribution of CVD in Denmark by individual age-specific mortality rates (Table V–4). Four separate age groups were used. With 132 cases in 9 regions comprising Denmark, there was no statistically significant variation from homogeneity for those age 45 to 54. Similarly, no significant variation (at our 1% level) was found for the 494 cases age 55 to 64 or the 1467 age 65 to 74. Only when we reach the 75 and over group, with 3319 cases in 169,000 population do we attain "statistical significance". The range in this last group was from 78 to 127% of the mean. Indeed most of the values in any age were close to the mean, and the individual high areas classed as "statistically significant" were *never* the same in any two age groups.

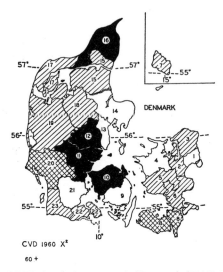

CVD 1960 X^2

60 +

Fig. V–7. Distribution of CVD deaths by county in Denmark (1960) against population age 60 and over, in "approximate χ-square" ranges, as in Fig. V–5. Data are in Appendix Table V–a–15

With this finding and those from county distributions in 1950 and 1960, it is safe to conclude that the CVD death distribution in Denmark does *not* depend on geography.

Scandinavian Medical Facilities and CVD Distributions. While in essence the distribution of stroke deaths can be considered quite uniform in Norway and Denmark (and in Sweden in 1960), the early Swedish distribution appeared irregular, even though not "focal". It seemed advisable therefore to see how the stroke deaths correlated with those of medical facilities (physicians, specialists, hospitals, hospital beds, hospital admissions). A relationship with population density was also sought. These findings are summarized in Table V–5, and we also can see there the correlations between the early and late CVD studies of Sweden and Denmark. Data are in the appropriate appendix tables.

For Norway and Denmark none of these factors showed any significant positive *or* negative correlation, and the early vs. late Danish strokes too were unrelated.

In Sweden in 1933 there were some interesting negative correlations with hospital admissions, population density, and all physicians (but not with urban

Table V–4. *Denmark — Distribution of CVD deaths among nine areas by age-specific mortality rates, expressed as percentages of the respective mean rates. Basic data are in Appendix Table V–a–20*

1961 cases/1960 pop.

Area	No.	Name	45—54	55—64	65—74	75 ≤
A	1	Copenhagen area	88.2	106.4	90.4	77.5
B	2—6	rest of Zealand	98.8	78.6	102.9	105.7
C	7	Bornholm	0	131.7	65.5	126.8*
D	8	Maribo	180.7*	90.1	96.2	99.5—
E	9+10	Funen	125.2	70.1	92.1	111.3**
F	11—14	E. Jutland	76.9	100.3	106.6	108.1
G	15—17	N. Jutland	120.9	91.8	99.95	119.9**
H	18—20	W. Jutland	109.8	120.0*	125.6**	106.9
I	21—23	S. Jutland	112.2	149.0**	95.8	101.7
Mean			100.0	100.0	100.0	100.0
rate per 10 M			2.21	10.21	46.07	196.00
N			132	494	1467	3319
% total CVD			2.43	9.10	27.01	61.11
Av. No. cases/area			15	55	163	369
population × 1000			598.0	483.9	318.4	169.3
χ^2			7.21	16.86	18.61	74.85
P			>0.30	>0.05	>0.02	<0.001

* = high of dubious significance (χ_a^2 2.0—4.0)
** = significantly high ($\chi_a^2 > 4.0$)

Table V–5. *Spearman rank-order correlations for distributions by county of cerebrovascular disease, expressed as "age-specific" mortality rates, with distributions of the following, also expressed in cases per unit population*

Subject	Norway 1946	Sweden 1933	Denmark 1950	Denmark 1960*
physicians	—0.06	—0.59 (t = —3.48)	—0.16	—0.26
urban physicians	—	+0.08	—	—
internists	—0.05	—	+0.06	+0.01
all specialists	—0.16	—	—	—
hospital beds	+0.22	—	+0.01	—0.16
number of hospitals	+0.26	—0.09	—	—
hospital admissions	+0.12	—0.36 (t = —1.87)	—	—
population density**	—0.12	—0.53 (t = —3.02)	+0.07	—0.06
CVD (1960)	—	+0.46 (t = 2.49)	+0.28	—
P = 0.05 r =	+0.40	+0.34	+0.36	+0.36 (1-tailed)
t =	±2.12	±2.07	±2.09	±2.09 (2-tailed)
P = 0.01 r =	+0.56	+0.48	+0.51	+0.51 (1-tailed)
t =	±2.58	±2.50	±2.53	±2.53 (2-tailed)

* against 1950 distributions
** persons/km², ranked from highest to lowest

physicians for these urban cases). There was also a significant (P < 0.05) positive association with the 1960 CVD distribution. Further elaboration of the interrelationships of medical facilities in Sweden for 1933 is described in Appendix Table V—a—17: hospital beds and admissions are almost unity (r = + 0.9). Population density is associated with hospital beds (or admissions) (r = + 0.5), and with all physicians (r = + 0.6) — but not with urban physicians (— 0.1) who are unrelated on *any* of these variables. Hospital beds (or admissions) are strongly related to the distribution of all physicians (r = + 0.7).

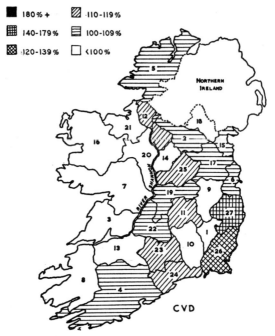

Fig. V—8. Distribution of CVD deaths by county in Ireland (1951—1955) against the population age 35 and over, in percentiles of the national mean mortality rate. Data are summarized in Table V—6, and detailed in Appendix Table V—a—18, from ACHESON (1960)

In terms of the strokes, there is some evidence then that the frequency of this diagnosis as a cause of death in Sweden in 1933 bears an inverse relationship to the adequacy of medical facilities. This may perhaps explain the much more homogeneous distribution for CVD deaths in 1960, when medical care would seem more widely available in this state-oriented system.

Ireland. To return to our investigation of the geographic distribution of CVD deaths, we have available the study of the Republic of Ireland reported by ACHESON (1960). His mortality rates were cited separately by sex and with County Boroughs distinct from the counties; the original data were no longer available [ACHESON, 1966 (2)]. The series was reconstructed from the published rates and consolidated by sex and region as shown in Appendix Table V—a—18 and summarized in Table V—6.

In Table V—6 is listed the distribution of CVD deaths in Ireland as percentages for each county of the (national) average annual mortality rate for CVD, based on population distributions age 35 and over. The national rate cited is 88 per 100,000 total population. Numbers 28 through 32 are the County Boroughs which have been included in the appropriate counties. The range of rates is from 55 to 165% of the national mean rate, but there are only two high areas (No. 26 and 27) beyond our criterion at 133 and 165% of the mean. The total χ-square values were 49 for 1200 males, 55 for 1400 females, and 97 for both sexes, while P = 0.01 at 45.6. Differences between the sexes were rather considerable, though the majority of rates were in the same direction (Appendix Table V—a—18).

Table V—6. *Distribution of Cerebrovascular Disease Deaths in Ireland, by County, 1951—1955*

County No.	% of mean rate	County No.	% of mean rate
1	82.2	15	106.8
2	107.9	16	58.9
3	78.4	17	106.0
4+28	109.8*	18	99.2
5	106.2	19	100.2
6+29+30	107.3*	20	78.6
7	82.7	21	93.5
8	84.7	22	105.0
9	82.6	23	116.2
10	85.6	24+32	113.8
11	110.3	25	116.7
12	110.7	26	132.8**
13+31	73.0	27	164.7**
14	54.9		
		Total: 100.0 = 88/100,000	

* = high of dubious significance (χ_a^2 2.0—4.0)
** = significantly high (χ_a^2 > 4.0)

With the small range for most regions and the variability between the sexes, I would be inclined to view this study too as indicating no major geographic features to the distribution of CVD in Eire.

United States. A careful study of the distribution of CVD deaths in the United States was published by BORHANI (1965). He limited consideration to whites age 35 to 64, as being most likely to have had correct diagnoses, and noted their distribution by state by means of age-adjusted annual mortality rates. Periods covered were 1949—51 and 1959—61, and he mapped these out as quartile ranges of the mortality rates, separately by sex and period.

Taking as the mean the midpoint between the second and third quartile, I have cited the average annual mortality rate by sex in 1959—61 for each state as its percentage of the respective national mean mortality rates. The findings are in Table V—7.

Immediately apparent is the tight range found for the individual states. For males the limits are 64% (Wyoming) to 168% (South Carolina) of the mean. Only

Table V-7. *United States — CVD deaths. Average annual age-adjusted mortality rates by state for white persons age 35—64, 1959—1961* (Borhani), *expressed as percentages of the national mean rate*

No.	State	Male	Female
1	Maine	107	100
2	New Hampshire	108	100
3	Vermont	83	117
4	Massachusetts	102	108
5	Rhode Island	92	102
6	Connecticut	101	101
7	New York	84	94
8	New Jersey	90	99.8
9	Pennsylvania	109.7	116
10	Ohio	103	111
11	Indiana	117	117
12	Illinois	102	105
13	Michigan	101	110
14	Wisconsin	105	109.8
15	Minnesota	95	108
16	Iowa	96	98
17	Missouri	96	94
18	N. Dakota	96	95
19	S. Dakota	87	82
20	Nebraska	82	84
21	Kansas	80	77
22	Delaware	94	81
23	Maryland	89	95
24	Virginia	114	96
25	W. Virginia	116	118
26	N. Carolina	140	112
27	S. Carolina	168	132
28	Georgia	148	126
29	Florida	104	90
30	Kentucky	118	113
31	Tennessee	131	110
32	Alabama	124	106
33	Mississippi	120	112
34	Arkansas	106	86
35	Louisiana	115	97
36	Oklahoma	99	83
37	Texas	98	86
38	Montana	82	80
39	Idaho	82	89
40	Wyoming	64	97
41	Colorado	71	83
42	New Mexico	92	93
43	Arizona	79	86
44	Utah	70	84
45	Nevada	116	135
46	Washington	100	108
47	Oregon	95	111
48	California	88	90
Total		100 = 53.7	100 = 41.9

four states (North Carolina, 140; South Carolina, 168; Georgia, 148, and Tennessee, 131) exceed our arbitrary 125% limit. The range in females is even smaller, being but 77% (Kansas) to 135% (Nevada). Now only three states are above our limit: South Carolina (132), Georgia (126), and Nevada (135).

In Fig. V—9 we can see pictorially the male CVD distributions. The deep South is the site of our "focus". What remnants there are of this "focus" in females are presented in Fig. V—10. The female CVD distribution especially strikes me as being essentially random, though we might look further to see if there is any reason there should be a concentration of strokes in the South.

Recalling our previous findings with Scandinavia, the obvious step was to compare CVD distributions with those of medical facilities. For simplicity I limited this to the distribution by state of non-federal physicians in 1962 (Fig. V—11, Appendix Table V—a—19).

It would certainly appear that where too many strokes were reported too few physicians were present.

A more formal approach was required however, and rank-order correlation tests run, the results of which are in Table V—8. Actually this linear coefficient did not attain statistical significance ($r = -0.2$) which would indicate either no association or a non-linear association between CVD and MD rates.

Table V—8. *CVD deaths in U. S. Correlations for distributions by state*

factors	r	r^2	t
Male 1949—1951 vs. 1959—1961	0.89	0.79	13.31
Female 1949—1951 vs. 1959—1961	0.60	0.36	5.08
Male vs. Female 1949—1951	0.58	0.34	4.81
Male vs. Female 1959—1961	0.69	0.48	6.48
Average of all four factors above vs. non-federal physicians 1962	—0.21	0.05	—1.44

$P = 0.10 \quad t = \pm 1.68$
$P = 0.01 \quad t = \pm 2.69$

Parenthetically, it is interesting that the male CVD deaths were much more highly related for 1950 vs. 1960 than were the sex distributions in either separate period, indicating to me that something other than geography is determining the distributions.

Since the maps suggested a reciprocal relationship between stroke death diagnosis and physicians, I then plotted for each state its own percentage of CVD mortality rate (males 1959—61) versus its own percentage of MD prevalence rate in physicians per 100,000 population. The results of this exercise are in Fig. V—12.

Several points are clear. First, I am confident a significant curvilinear regression line could be fitted to these data; this I will leave to others. Of more import, when we look at the upper right quadrant representing high stroke and high physician rates, it, like Hubbard's cupboard, is practically bare. Some low rates are found

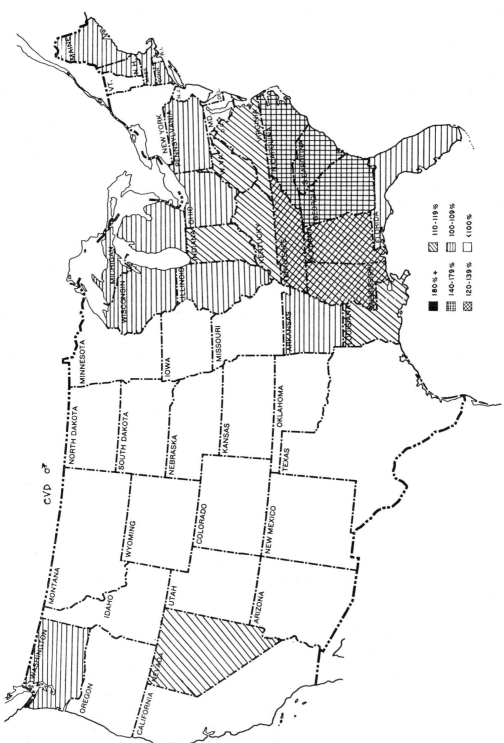

Fig. V–9. Distribution of CVD deaths by state in the United States (1959–1961) for white males age 35—64, in percentiles of the national mean mortality rate. Data are in Table V–7, from BORHANI (1965)

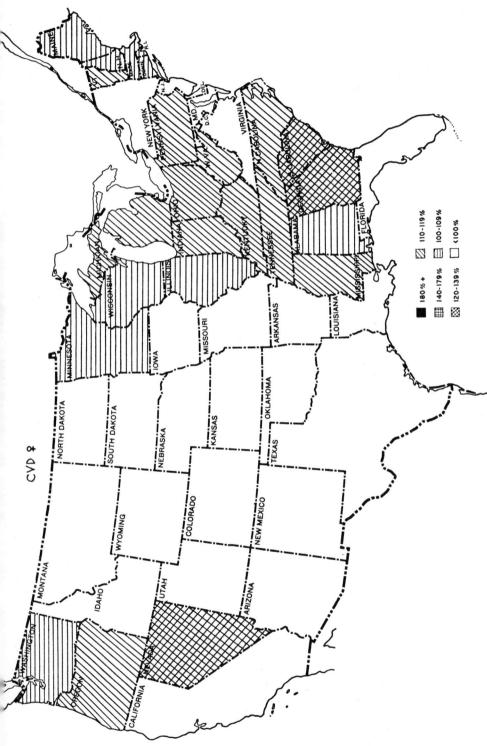

Fig. V–10. Distribution of CVD deaths by state in the United States (1959—1961) for white females age 35—64, in percentiles of the national mean mortality rate. Data are in Table V–7, from BORHANI (1965)

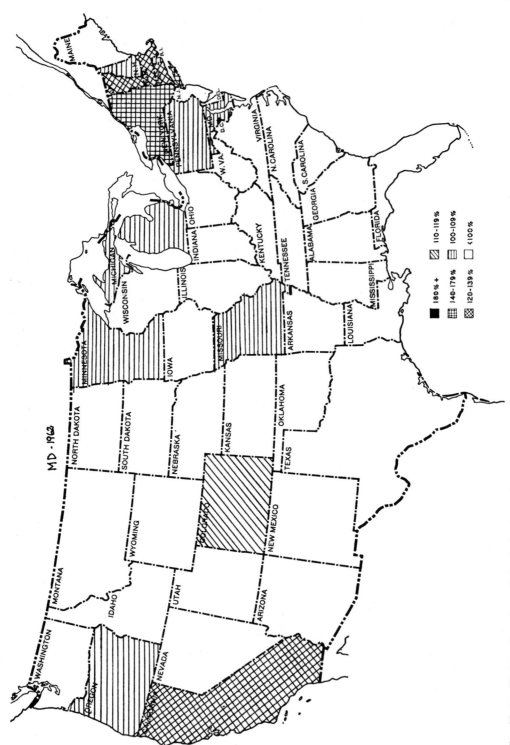

Fig. V–11. Distribution of non-federal physicians by state in the United States (1962), as percentiles of national mean prevalence rate. Data are

for strokes where physicians are high. Then, a fair number of rates cluster about
the mean intercept of both stroke and MD. Where physicians are few, variability
of stroke rates is the most pronounced.

Most importantly though, in *all* the areas where strokes exceeded some 115%
of the national mean, physicians were represented at a frequency of some 80%
or less of the national mean! Therefore, high stroke death rate reports in the United
States could be considered an indicator of a scarcity of physicians, and, by inference, of medical facilities in general. As also with Scandinavia, I take this as a
reflection of poor *reporting*. Where medical care is limited, common and popular

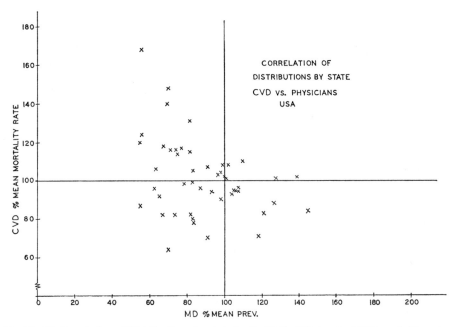

Fig. V–12. Correlation of distributions by state in the United States for CVD mortality rates
and physician prevalence rates, each expressed as percentages of the respective national mean
rates. CVD cases are white males age 35—64 (1959—1961), from Table V–7; physicians (1962)
from Appendix Table V–a–19

causes of death would be expected to be cited more than the true frequencies
warrant, while those of a more sophisticated nature would be underrepresented.
By no means can one infer from these data that CVD deaths themselves are
inversely related to physicians. While we would like to believe our ministrations
do indeed increase survival, there is really no solid evidence to this point. The
course of CVD is discussed in Chapter XI.

Considering the vastness of the subcontinent which is the United States, with
almost 200 million people in 3 million square miles looked after by a quarter
million physicians, and with the extreme diversity of the populations therein,
I think it is almost astounding to find such minimal differences among the states
for the distribution of CVD deaths in the white citizens. Add to that the evidence

that links high CVD rates and low physician rates, and I believe that the distribution of CVD deaths within the United States must be considered to be essentially homogeneous.

We can of course inspect the Scandinavian CVD data in the same fashion. In Fig. V–13, I think one can see that the results are quite similar. *Most* of the high rate areas are indeed concentrated where physicians are sparse. The Swedish data (1933) seem more scattered, and are drawn with open circles, but generally seem to behave in similar fashion. The MD rates for Sweden referred to were the urban MD, which had been found above to show no significant linear correlation,

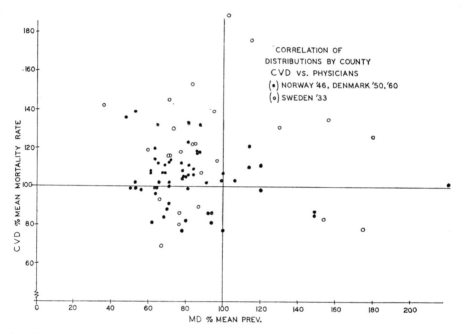

Fig. V–13. Correlation of distributions by county in Scandinavia for CVD mortality rates and physician prevalence rates, each expressed as percentages of the respective national mean rates. Findings for Norway (1946) and Denmark (1950, 1960) are plotted as solid circles, those for Sweden (1933) as open circles. Data are in appropriate Chapter V Appendix Tables

unlike the distributions of other medical facilities. Thus even these urban physician rates bear *some* inverse relation to CVD death reports.

References

ACHESON, R. M. 2, 6
ADIN 10
Almindelige Danske Laege-
  forening 14
ALSING 15, 16
BORHANI 36
Central Statistics Office 55

Kungl. Medicinalstyrelsen
  186
KURTZKE 189—194
LAURSSEN 198
SODELAND 333
Statistisk Sentralbyrå
  338—340

Statistiska Centralbyrån
  341—346
det Statistiske Departement
  347
Sundhedsstyrelsen 349, 350
U. S. Bureau of the Census
  370—373

Chapter VI

CVD-Major Divisions and Subarachnoid Hemorrhage

Thus far we have used the artificial device of classing all cerebrovascular disease as an entity. In this fashion it would appear we are dealing with a disorder that is strikingly related to age, but which otherwise seems to affect equally both sexes in all lands and in all regions of the lands. The "lands" of course are limited to those we have looked at, and "all regions" is somewhat of an exaggeration for effect. But thus far any evidence suggesting a link of CVD with the environment, the macroclimate, is discouragingly lacking. However the totality could well incorporate entities which either act in opposite directions or are masked by their small numbers in reference to the whole. It is therefore in order to look at the components of "stroke".

Relative Frequency of Types of CVD. As covered in Chapter II, our basic divisions of CVD arise from the ISC mortality code, and are subarachnoid hemorrhage (SAH) (Code 330); cerebral hemorrhage (CbH) (331); cerebral thrombosis-embolism (Cb Thr-Emb) (332); and "other CVD" (334). To these categories we are limited for data from one of our main sources of information, mortality statistics. With our other resources, hospital series and population surveys-especially the former, this skeleton can be fleshed out. For our preliminary view however we shall keep to the ISC codes.

In Appendix Table VI–a–1 are the average annual age-adjusted mortality rates for categories of CVD. The rates are from the same 18 countries discussed in Chapter IV which appeared to me to be of adequate medical and reporting standards. They are among the 33 presented by GOLDBERG (1962) with data cited by STALLONES (1965), wherein all rates pertain to the 1951—1958 period and are age-standardized to the US population. Considering the relative uniformity of the total CVD rates (see Table IV–1), there are very wide variations among the components. Cerebral hemorrhage, for example, ranges from 14 cases per 100,000 population in Belgium to 101 in Finland. However, I have taken the weighted mean of these countries for each category, and from the mean we have the first line of Table VI–1.

In this table the relative proportions are listed as percentages of the whole within the major ISC classes. In those from mortality statistics, we also see the frequencies for Denmark in 1956—1960, for England and Wales in 1960 (DU BOULAY, 1965) and in 1949 [WYLIE, 1962 (1)], and for the United States in 1948 and 1958 (WYLIE, 1961).

SAH would seem to average some 3% of CVD cases from mortality data, and as a group would obviously be lost from view when we look at all strokes together. Whether cerebral hemorrhage deaths are more numerous than thrombosis, as in the weighted mean, Denmark, USA, England (1949); or less numerous, as in

England (1960), is difficult to decide. The trend would appear to be toward fewer reports of cerebral hemorrhage. This topic gets somewhat complex, and for its consideration a separate chapter (X) has been reserved. "Other" CVD as an entity does seem to be cited less frequently in most of the more recent works, but not for

Table VI−1. *Percentage frequency, types of CVD*

Source	Year	SAH (330)	Cb. H. (331)	Cb. Thr-E. (332)	Other (334)	Total (300-334)	N
A — from mortality statistics							
Weighted mean 18 countries	1951—1958	2.8	54.2	29.2	13.8	100.0	—
Denmark	1956—1960	1.5	69.5	18.7	10.3	100.0	26394
„ males	1956—1960	1.3	68.1	19.5	11.1	100.0	12230
„ females	1956—1960	1.7	70.8	17.9	9.6	100.0	14164
England-Wales (DU BOULAY)	1960	4.5	38.0	48.9	8.5	99.9	76220
„ males	1960	4.2	37.7	49.2	8.9	100.0	31006
„ females	1960	4.7	38.3	48.8	8.3	100.1	45214
England-Wales (WYLIE, 1962)	1949	2.2	53.8	39.1	5.0	100.1	—
USA (white) (WYLIE)	1948	1.8	68.2	16.1	13.9	100.0	—
USA (white) (WYLIE)	1958	3.0	58.9	29.0	9.0	99.9	—
B — from hospital series							
New York (GROCH)	1956—1960	5.0	6.9	79.4	8.9	100.2	667
Middlesex, England (CARTER, 1963)	1952—1961	9.7	38.9	51.4	0.0	100.0	1402
C — from population surveys							
Framingham, Mass. (KANNEL)	1949—1962	18	4	78	0	100	90
Rochester, Minn. (KURLAND, 1967)	1957	9	16	50	25	100	64
Middlesex, Conn. (EISENBERG)	1957—1958	— 36 —		50	14	100	191
Goulburn, Australia (WALLACE)	1962—1964	6	17	72	5	100	155
C-weighted mean, 4 studies		12.4*	15.8*	61.6	10.2	100.0	500

* adjusted for Middlesex

England. There are no compelling reasons from *these* data to consider changing the proportions indicated by the 18 countries in the 1950's.

Only two large hospital series are cited. While they were not chosen with a view to bringing out discrepancies, they are obviously different. I do not believe we can determine "true" proportions for stroke components from hospital data. The English series of Carter (1963) looks similar to his own country's mortality data, but that from Bellevue Hospital by GROCH (1961) is unlike any mortality series.

We should obtain our best information on the "true" proportions of stroke-types from population surveys. Listed are the four which speak to this point, all of which have been mentioned in Chapter IV. The Framingham study of KANNEL (1965) is part of an ongoing survey primarily aimed at cardiovascular disease. The Rochester material of KURLAND (1967) and the Connecticut study by EISENBERG (1964) were oriented toward CVD. WALLACE (1967) performed a detailed survey of stroke in Goulburn, Australia. From among these four works we have figures quite as discrepant as from among the mortality series. The weighted averages of these four though do give us our best available evidence on the relative frequencies of the various types of stroke in the general population, during the past 10 years.

Table VI−2. *Age-distribution, percentage frequency for deaths due to subarachnoid hemorrhage versus all other cerebrovascular diseases*

Age group	Subarachnoid		All other CVD		Total CVD		
	(a)	(b)	(a)	(b)	(a)	(b)	(c)
0—24	3.2	7.2	0.1	0.1	0.2	0.2	0.3
25—44	14.7	20.4	0.6	0.4	1.3	0.7	1.0
45—64	48.0	44.3	14.5	11.1	15.9	11.6	16.7
65—74	20.4	20.4	28.1	28.0	27.7	27.8	32.0
75 ≤	13.6	7.7	56.8	60.4	54.9	59.6	49.9
Total	99.9	100.0	100.1	100.0	100.0	99.9	99.9
N	3447	402	72,775	25,992	76,222	26,394	3135

(a) England-Wales 1960 (DU BOULAY)
(b) Denmark 1956—1960
(c) Denmark 1950

In this fashion we can *estimate* that at present approximately 12% of all CVD will be SAH, 16% cerebral hemorrhage, 62% cerebral thrombosis, and 10% "other or ill-defined" CVD.

On the assumption that the annual incidence of CVD is about 200 cases per 100,000 (and 207 was the rate observed in the Middlesex, Rochester material), the average annual incidence for types of CVD should then be about 25 for SAH, 32 for cerebral hemorrhage, 123 for thrombosis-embolism, and 20 for "other" CVD. My guess is that the SAH figure is somewhat too high, and I think the first two figures are more likely some 20 for SAH and 40 for hemorrhage. PAKARINEN (1967) in Helsinki found an incidence rate of 16 for SAH and about 32 for cerebral hemorrhage. SJÖSTRÖM (1967) reported incidence rates of 15 for SAH, 107 for hemorrhage, 62 for thrombosis-embolism, and 40 for "other" CVD. These were rates based on hospitalized patients in a large region of Sweden in 1964; half the patients died and about a third of the deaths were autopsied. As will be discussed later, I think the cerebral hemorrhage figure is grossly inflated at the expense of thrombosis.

These proportions would appear much different from those of mortality rates. Obviously the latter are based on those who die, and also obviously the fatality rates are not the same for all. While we shall cover in more detail the various case-fatality rates below (Chapter XI) let us now assign rather arbitrary values for early deaths in these categories. If early fatalities comprise 30% of SAH, 90% of hemorrhage, 40% of thrombosis, and 60% of "others", we would expect from the observed population frequencies to find mortality statistics to be in the order of the following: for SAH, 8%; hemorrhage, 30%; thrombosis, 50%; and "other CVD", 12%. The mortality data of England-Wales for 1960 at least are quite close to these proportions.

Subarachnoid Hemorrhage — Mortality Data. With the small fraction of CVD provided by SAH, little can be inferred about its behavior from the totality of

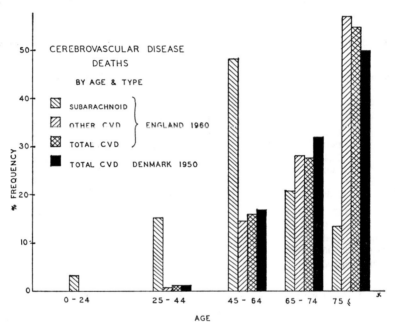

Fig. VI–1. Percentage frequency distribution by age for SAH deaths vs. other CVD deaths in England (1960), and compared with all CVD deaths in Denmark (1950). Data in Table VI–2

stroke. When we segregate this entity from the remainder, as in Table VI–2, we see the markedly different age-distribution for SAH. The median age of SAH deaths in Denmark is 56 years, which is 20 years less than that for the remainder of CVD (Appendix Table VI–a–2). In England too (DU BOULAY, 1965), we find this same discrepancy, the extent of which may be more obvious when we graph the percentages (Fig. VI–1).

Average annual age-specific mortality rates for SAH and all other CVD deaths in Denmark in 1956—1960 are plotted in Fig. VI–2 (data in Appendix Table VI–a–3). We include for reference the US-England CVD line of Chapter IV. The SAH mortality rates rise from 0.2 per 100,000 at age 0 to 14 to 1.9 by age 35 to 39. But the increase thereafter is slight, reaching a peak of 5.8 at age 70 to 74, and possibly declining thereafter. This is a grossly different pattern from the remainder of stroke.

Similar findings are apparent in the Netherlands (GIEL, 1965). In Fig. VI—3, we have the annual age-specific rates for SAH deaths in that country for two periods, 1950—1954 and 1958—1962. Both fit well within the confidence limits for the Danish death rates. For either the total rates or those of any given age, the sex-ratio is practically unity (Appendix Table VI—a—4). Other information on male-female ratios for all SAH is in Appendix Table VI—a—12, and would

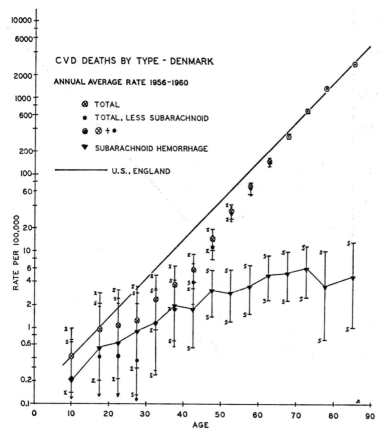

Fig. VI—2. Average annual age-specific mortality rates for SAH vs. remainder of CVD in Denmark (1956—1960), in cases per 100,000 population, with 95% confidence limits on the rates. Heavy solid line represents US-England CVD deaths. Data are in Appendix Table VI—a—3

indicate variations to either side. Danish age-specific mortality rates however with rather small numbers would generally indicate a female preponderance (Appendix Table VI—a—13).

Therefore SAH would seem to provide about 3 deaths annually per 100,000 population, with a lesser number in the young and but slightly higher frequencies in the older ages. No information on the components of SAH is available from mortality data, and our population surveys too fail us in this regard. For further evaluation therefore we turn to hospital series.

4*

SAH — **Clinical Data.** A massive cooperative study of SAH has recently been completed. Without a doubt this will be the standard for comparison for years. The study was reported *seriatim* in the Journal of Neurosurgery volumes 24 and 25 of 1966, and the authors of each paper are so identified in the references to this chapter. This, the Cooperative Study of Intracranial Aneurysms and Subarachnoid Hemorrhage, involved 19 university centers in the United States and one in

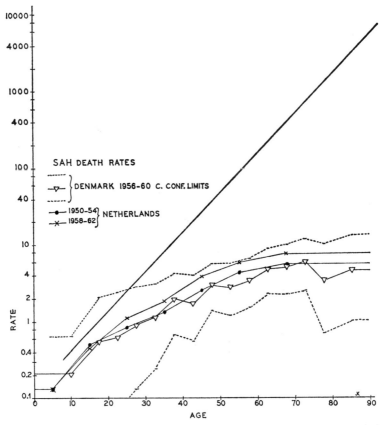

Fig. VI–3. Age-specific average annual mortality rates for SAH deaths in the Netherlands (1950—1954 and 1958—1962), superimposed on the Danish SAH rates and confidence limits from Fig. VI–2. Heavy line represents US-England CVD deaths. Data for the Netherlands are in Appendix Table VI–a–4, from GIEL (1965)

England, and between 1958 and 1965 studied over 6000 cases of aneurysm, arteriovenous malformation (AVM), and/or non-traumatic subarachnoid hemorrhage. "Contributors and Centers" are listed by SAHS et al. (J. Neurosurg. **24**, 779, not cited in my references).

In Chapter II SAH was classified by cause as that with aneurysm, with AVM, with hypertension (HT) and/or arteriosclerosis (AS), with miscellaneous states, and with none discernable (= idiopathic). Table VI–3 indicates the proportions of each which were found in the Cooperative Study (LOCKSLEY), and similar figures from two moderately large individual studies not part of the former: TRUMPY's work (1967) from Norway, and AF BJÖRKESTEN's (1965) from Finland. We can see that half the SAH in the Cooperative Study were associated with congenital (berry) aneurysm and 6% with AVM; less than 1% had both lesions. HT and/or AS was associated with the bleed in 15%, and a variety of states with SAH in 6%. In 22% no lesion could be demonstrated after complete study. The figures of AF BJÖRKESTEN are quite similar; general vascular disease was not mentioned. In his study, only those with complete angiography of both carotids and both vertebrals were included. With this point we would appear to be able to explain the discrepant findings of TRUMPY in whose series half the bleeds had no demonstrable cause, and few had complete angiography.

SAH — Aneurysm. SAH in general was shown above to be a disorder with a peak in mid-adult life but with a notable frequency in the young and throughout the senium. SAH with aneurysm too follows this pattern (Fig. VI–4). There is a significant age-difference by sex. The mean age in males was 46.8 and in females 55.5 (Appendix Table VI–a–5). This difference, as pointed out by LOCKSLEY (1966), is not attributable to population variations by age and sex. In fact there are still other unexpected sex differences in aneurysm, as we shall see.

The same frequencies for age are apparent in Fig. VI–5 from Maida Vale Hospital in London, as reported by DU BOULAY (1965) in a paper far more broad than its title would indicate. In this figure the bleeding aneurysms are compared with his series of brain tumor cases, and are seen to be the same (Appendix Table VI–a–6). Includ-

Table VI–3. *Major causes of spontaneous subarachnoid hemorrhage (SAH): (A) from Cooperative Study* (LOCKSLEY), *(B) from Bergen, Norway* (TRUMPY), *and (C) from Helsinki, Finland* (AF BJÖRKESTEN)

Cause	Percentage Frequency		
	(A)	(B)	(C)
Aneurysm only	51	32	65
AVM only	6	6	5
HT and/or AS	15	7	—
HT only	5	—	—
HT and AS	8	—	—
AS only	2	—	—
Idiopathic	22	53*	15
Miscellaneous	6	3	15
Total	100	100	100
N	4880	229	113

* Only $1/3$ had bilateral carotid angiograms, and no autopsies done. AVM = arteriovenous malformation; HT = hypertension; AS = arteriosclerosis

ed here too are distributions for age at ictus for the more common CVD which are comparable to the frequencies for age at death in all strokes, as in Fig. VI–1.

Locations of aneurysms are cited in Table VI–4 from several sources. In the Cooperative Study the internal carotid region was the most common site, and better than half of these originated on the posterior communicating artery. The large majority of anterior cerebral aneurysms, which were $1/3$ of the total, were found on the anterior communicating. Middle cerebral aneurysms, proximal or distal, were present in $1/5$ of cases, and those of basilar-vertebral system, including the posterior cerebrals, were uncommon. McKISSOCK's London experience (1964) was generally quite comparable; though he was part of the Cooperative Study, half his cases reported here could not have been not included in the Study, and the similarities are not explicable by the same cases being counted twice. The locations in the much smaller series of TRUMPY and AF BJÖRKESTEN were in moderate

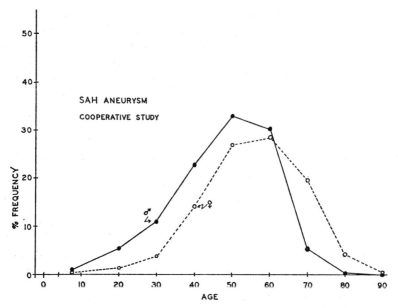

Fig. VI–4. Percentage frequency distribution by age and sex for SAH due to aneurysm. Data are in Appendix Table VI–a–5, from the Cooperative Study [LOCKSLEY, 1966 (1, 2)]

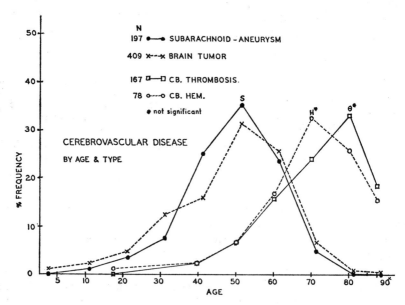

Fig. VI–5. Percentage frequency distribution by age for hospital cases of SAH due to aneurysm and of brain tumor, compared with population survey cases of cerebral thrombosis and hemorrhage. Data are in Appendix Table VI–a–6 for the hospital series, from DU BOULAY (1965), and in the next chapter in Appendix Table VII–a–3, from KURLAND (1967) and EISENBERG (1964)

Table VI – 4. *Summary for locations of single aneurysms from (A) Cooperative Study* (Locksley); *(B) London, England* (McKissock); *(C) Bergen, Norway* (Trumpy); *and (D) Helsinki, Finland* (af Björkesten)

Site	(A)			(B)			(C)	(D)
	M	F	Σ	M	F	Σ	Σ	Σ
	(percentages)							
Internal carotid	29.8	49.8	41.2	30.1	39.4	35.5	23.8	26.0
(post. communic.)	(18.8)	(29.7)	(25.0)	(21.4)	(33.6)	(28.4)	—	(23.5)
Anterior cerebral	44.7	25.2	33.5	42.5	31.6	36.1	38.1	30.2
(ant. communic.)	(38.3)	(20.3)	(28.0)	(39.5)	(28.0)	(32.8)	—	(24.4)
Middle cerebral	19.1	20.3	19.8	21.9	24.3	23.3	31.8	33.6
Posterior circuit*	6.3	4.7	5.4	5.6	4.8	5.2	6.4	10.1
Total	99.9	100.0	99.9	100.1	100.1	100.1	100.1	99.9
N	1135	1537	2672	608	847	1455	63	119
Cases with multiple aneurysms	—	—	20%	12%	19%	15%	16%	30%

* Includes post. cerebral

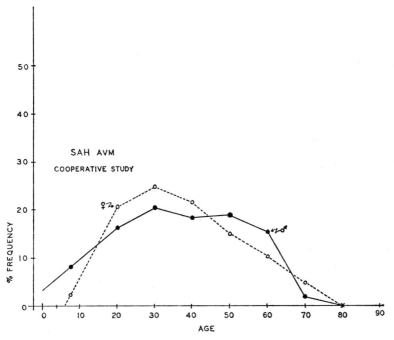

Fig. VI – 6. Percentage frequency distribution by age and sex for SAH due to AVM. Data are in Appendix Table VI – a – 5, from the Cooperative Study [Locksley, 1966 (1, 2)]

agreement. Some 20% of aneurysms were multiple. More detail from the Cooperative Study is provided in Appendix Table VI–a–7.

Looking once more at the sex differences, we see that the females were not only older but also more numerous. The male/female ratio was 0.7 in the Cooperative

Study and in London. This too is beyond expected population differences. But we also have a very strange difference in *location*. Internal carotid aneurysms were much less common in males and anterior cerebral aneurysms much more common. This is true of these vessels in whole or in part (e. g. the communicating vessels). Middle cerebral and posterior circuit aneurysms however were equal. Though somewhat less striking, the same differences were seen in the London series. I have no logical answer for any of these variations, nor for the right-sided preponderance which was *also* present.

SAH — AVM. The age-distribution with arteriovenous malformation is drawn in Fig. VI–6, from data in Appendix Table VI–a–5 which too was abstracted

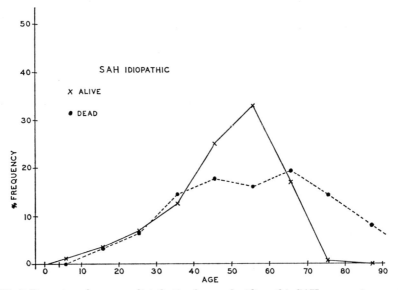

Fig. VI–7. Percentage frequency distribution by age for idiopathic SAH, comparing survivors with fatalities. Data are in Appendix Table VI–a–11, from the Cooperative Study [LOCKSLEY, 1966 (4)]

from the Cooperative Study. It is obvious this is a much younger group. The mean age as 38 for (happily) males *and* females. The M/F ratio of 1.2 is not too discrepant from unity in these 272 cases.

AVM are discovered because they either bleed or act as focal lesions. Age distributions of AVM without SAH suggested they were a somewhat older group than those with SAH, according to PERRET (1966) of the Cooperative Study (Appendix Table VI–a–8). Mean age was 35 for those with and 38 for those without SAH. The figures here differ from previous tables, as was true of many parts of the Cooperative Study report, since varying criteria determined inclusion in any given list. In addition precisely the opposite age variation was found in SVEIN's series (1965) from the Mayo Clinic (Appendix Table VI–a–9) where the bleeders were 28 and non-bleeders 25 years old. Therefore there seems to be little intrinsic difference in age for the manifestations of AVM.

SAH — Other. Age distributions of SAH associated with hypertension, arteriosclerosis, or both are set forth in Appendix Table VI–a–10. The hypertensives were some 55 years of age on the average, those with both about 60, and those with arteriosclerosis, age 64. Males were generally somewhat more numerous than females in each category. The Cooperative Study was the source of these data.

The group of patients with SAH in whom no lesion was demonstrable after complete angiographic and clinical study, or at autopsy, and who had no associated medical illness, I have classed as "idiopathic" SAH. Their ages are not dissimilar from those for all SAH, the mean being some 50 years. Fig. VI—7 shows the distributions for 286 survivors and the 62 who succumbed with idiopathic SAH within three months. The mean age for the latter was 55, vs. 48 for the others. Of course these cases could be instances of hamartomas, or minute vascular malformations (MARGOLIS, 1961); even at autopsy such lesions cannot be ruled out.

SAH — Integration. Since we have little direct information, any estimate on the population frequency of SAH cases would be just that. Still we can see what our material does suggest. Mortality rates, we may recall, were about 1.8 per 100,000 near age 30, some 4 near age 50, and 6 near age 70, from the Danish series. Most SAH of the young are AVM, those in the middle years aneurysm and idiopathic, and those in the older ages associated with vascular disease. Each entity, as we shall see, has its own case-fatality rate, and within each there is an additional positive association between age and death. As we did previously for types of CVD, arbitrary case-fatality rates for SAH at different ages can be set down: for young adults, 20%; at age 50, 40%; and at age 70, 70%. In this manner, population frequencies (annual incidence rates) would be about 9 or 10 cases of SAH per 100,000 for all ages after childhood (9, 10, and 9 from the above calculations), and for any age-group therein. Thus SAH would *seem* to be about equally prevalent throughout adult life, and the rise with age on mortality rates a resultant of an increasing case-fatality rate.

We mentioned above the survey of PAKARINEN (1967) in Helsinki. He discussed some 600 cases of SAH found between 1954 and 1961. Age specific annual incidence rates rose from some 1 per 100,000 in childhood to nearly 30 per 100,000 by age 40, with but little change thereafter. Thus his adult rates are about three times as high as those just calculated, which were based on an average mortality rate of 3 per 100,000. We have estimated earlier in this chapter that SAH mortality rates should be about 8 per 100,000. PAKARINEN's was indeed about 8 and his incidence was 16. This study then would provide some validation for our higher estimate, as well as further supporting the relatively even frequency of SAH throughout adult life. He too noted a relationship of fatality rates with age.

The interrelationships of cause and effect in SAH may be summarized as in Fig. VI—8. In the left-hand bar we represent lesions which may cause SAH. These are from the bottom, hypertension/arteriosclerosis; AVM; aneurysm; brain tumor (other than AVM); and other medical conditions. The height of the bar indicates the *estimated* relative frequency of each condition as it is encountered in medical practice. Hypertension and/or arteriosclerosis, as well as "other medical diseases" are left open-ended.

Now for each type of lesion, the signs which bring the patient under medical observation may be classed as (1) evidence of mass lesion, (2) evidence of bleed or SAH, and (3) other phenomena. For each lesion, the relative frequency of these presenting signs is designated as the proportion of the lesion-bar it occupies, and again they are clinical estimates. Mass is vertical-lined, SAH is open, and "other" is wide diagonal-lined. For example most brain tumors present as space-occupying lesions and very few as subarachnoid hemorrhage, while the opposite situation holds for aneurysm. With AVM the proportions of each are relatively equal. More patients with HT/AS will show SAH than evidence of intracranial mass lesion, but most of course will show neither.

From each lesion-bar we then take that proportion of cases represented by SAH to the right-hand block, which represents all SAH. This block builds vertically to

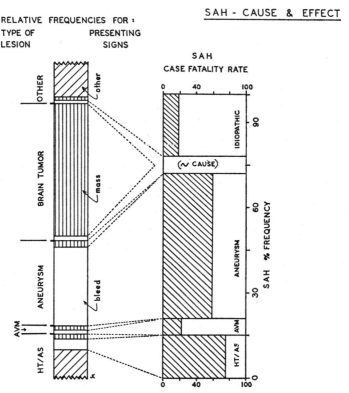

Fig. VI–8. SAH — cause and effect. The left-hand bar represents proportions of causative lesions with their own respective proportions of presenting signs. That fraction of each which is SAH is taken to the right hand block which builds vertically to 100% SAH. Horizontally in each SAH-cause block is its own case-fatality rate. See text for further explanation

100% by adding together the separate causes of SAH, with the frequencies found in the Cooperative Study (Table VI–3): 15% HT/AS, 6% AVM, and 51% aneurysm; the 6% "other SAH" are derived from tumor plus other medical conditions, and the 22% idiopathic SAH complete the block for SAH.

Within each SAH-cause block, we also denote the respective case-fatality rates, which are covered in Chapter XI. Aneurysm is near 60%, AVM and idiopathic near 20%, HT/AS near 75%, and the "other" group varies depending on the cause of the lesion producing SAH.

References

CVD divisions

CARTER 54
DU BOULAY 87
EISENBERG 93
GOLDBERG 125
GROCH 131, 132
KANNEL 169, 170
KURLAND 188
PAKARINEN 282
SJÖSTRÖM 328
WALLACE 379
WYLIE 396, 397

SAH

AF BJÖRKESTEN 12
CRAWFORD 64
DU BOULAY 87
EISENBERG 93
GIEL 121
KNOWLER* 179
KURLAND 188
LOCKSLEY* 203—206
MARGOLIS 214
McCORMICK* 227
McKISSOCK 233—237

NISHIOKA* 270
PAKARINEN 282
PERRET* 291, 292
SAHS* 313—315
SARNER 316, 317
SVEIN 352
TRUMPY 366
UIHLEIN 369
WALTON 380

* papers of the Cooperative
  Study

Chapter VII

Cerebral Hemorrhage and Thrombosis

Cerebral Hemorrhage. In the previous chapter we considered the relative frequencies of cerebral hemorrhage and thrombosis within both mortality and incidence studies. We estimated from the latter that mortality statistics should provide at present about 30% of CVD deaths as cerebral hemorrhage and about 50% as thrombosis-embolism. We saw however that observed frequencies were quite discrepant. Further they were extremely variable, so much so that I think *any* differentiation between hemorrhage and thrombosis based on mortality data is hazardous.

Notwithstanding these major reservations, let us inspect some further detail on cerebral hemorrhage, thrombosis, and "other" deaths. Percentage frequency distributions for the three types and the total in Denmark 1956—1960 are in Appendix Table VII—a—1. The median age is 78 years for *all* the subdivisions. Age-specific annual average mortality rates from this series (Appendix Table VII—a—2) are drawn in Fig. VII—1. All three entities provide a similar straight-line logarithmic relationship. At a given age the hemorrhage: thrombosis: "other" mortality rate ratio is about 10:3:1. The similar trend lines would suggest either three separate entities with the same age-spectrum, or consistent diagnostic bias, and I believe there is some truth to the latter. Similar findings are seen in Sweden (LARSSON, 1967), where however the ratios are about 10:5:4.

Percentage frequency distributions for the two entities from the population surveys of KURLAND (1967) and EISENBERG (1964) suggest that hemorrhage occurs at a somewhat younger age than thrombosis, the means being 73 and 75, and the medians a bit older. However there is no statistically significant difference between the two (Appendix Table VII—a—3). The two curves were drawn in Fig. VI—5 where they were compared with SAH age distributions.

Age-specific annual mortality rates for cerebral hemorrhage in Göteborg, Sweden indicate the same type of rise with age (Appendix Table VII—a—4). Since this series of AURELL (1964) refers only to deaths in the general hospital, the absolute rates are low. Adding in however the deaths from the chronic hospital, we have in 1948—1949 an annual mortality rate of 19 to 24 per 100,000 general population, depending on whether we include the "late deaths" which provide the higher figure (67 to 84 cases a year in 353,991 population). In 1960—1961, the general mortality rate for cerebral hemorrhage is similarly 20 to 25 per 100,000 (84.5 to 102.5 cases a year in 414,466 population). Allowing for the fact that not all deaths, even in Sweden, will occur in hospital, we see that these annual mortality rates are probably not very discrepant from the 30% of CVD deaths we have posited previously as attributable to cerebral hemorrhage, and certainly closer to this figures than the much higher one currently cited for cerebral hemorrhage in Scandinavia. Despite the author's contention, I find no significant difference between any or all the age-specific rates for the two periods. Age-specific incidence rates from the population surveys mentioned also indicate a steep rise in cerebral hemorrhage with age. Numbers are so small though that I have too little confidence even to draw them (Appendix Table VII—a—5).

Sex ratios in cerebral hemorrhage are 0.84 male/female from Danish mortality rates and 0.89 from EISENBERG's incidence rates (Appendix Table VII—a—6). Two European hospital series (FELGER, 1961 and ZIELKE, 1964) provide ratios

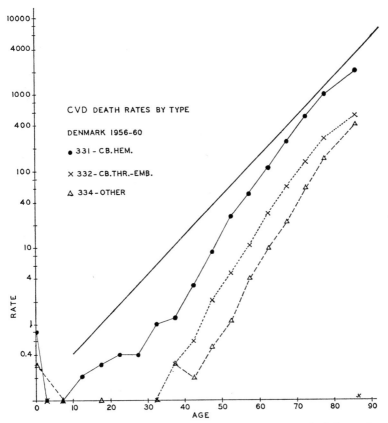

Fig. VII—1. Age specific average annual mortality rates for cerebral hemorrhage (331), cerebral thrombosis-embolism (332), and "other CVD" (334) in Denmark (1956—1960). Data from Appendix Table VII—a—2

of 1.3 and 0.7 respectively. The individual age-specific mortality rates vary irregularly about 1.00 in Denmark (Appendix Table VII—a—7). Keep in mind that sex ratios based on total population distributions tend to inflate the female proportion. "True" ratios should be determined not only from population-based rates rather than numbers of cases, but also from age-specific rather than total rates. Such requirements of course seriously restrict our sources of information, since we also need a goodly number of cases to provide stable rates and ratios. Only when, as in the SAH Cooperative Study, one subgroup stands out as different from the remainder in sex frequencies can we really rely on data distant in nature from our optimum. The best evidence for cerebral hemorrhage then would suggest a male/female ratio which is near unity.

Cerebral Thrombosis-Embolism. In clinical practice, even if not in mortality data, the bulk of our "strokes" are cerebral infarcts resulting from thrombo-embolic occlusive cerebral vascular disease. From the weighted mean of the population surveys already discussed, this group was seen to comprise 62% of CVD cases. Age-specific incidence rates are cited in Table VII–1. They would look similar to the CVD mortality curves previously drawn. Thus the striking relationship between age and CVD is seen also in this category. Strokes have been described

Table VII–1. *Age-specific annual incidence rates, cases per 100,000 population for cerebral thrombosis, from population surveys in USA*

Age group	(1) Middlesex Conn.	(2) Rochester Minn.	(3) (1) and (2)	(6) Framingham Mass.
< 35	0	0	0	—
35—39 40—44	0	20	5	— 13
45—49 50—54	40	70	48	78
55—59 60—64	180	180	180	215
65—69 70—74	380	250	350	—
75—79 80—84	1170	1040	1140	
85 ≤	2900	1390	2520	—
Average	80*	80	80	—
N	91	32	123	55

* Age-adjusted to US population.
(1) EISENBERG (1964); (2) KURLAND (1967); (6) KANNEL (1965).

in childhood but rarely. WISOFF (1961) could find thrombotic occlusion of cerebral blood vessels reported in but 31 children ranging from infancy to age 16. Additions to 1967 are few (DAVIE). In none of these was arteriosclerosis present; most of those with a defined cause were the resultant of congenital anomalies of blood vessels with dissecting aneurysm underlying the intraluminal thrombus. At The New York Hospital WELLS (1961) had only 77 patients under age 50 who were diagnosed as having cerebral thrombosis; of these, 55 were aged 40 to 49 and 12 were 30 to 39. 42% were hypertensive. Only one of the group died in the acute illness. HILTNER (1964) in Leipzig could collect only 89 patients with CVD under age 50 over a 15 year period, of whom 64% were hypertensive. At Bellevue Hospital, 56 patients with cerebral thrombosis, or some 6% of the total, were found to be age 50 or less (LOUIS, 1966), and 43 of these were in the 41 to 50 decade. Hypertension was present in 59%; 22% were overtly and 20% latently diabetic at the time of the stroke. In only four patients were there no associated factors of hypertension, diabetes, hypercholesterolemia, or other medical diseases to which the thrombosis could be attributed. In only one instance was the stroke the cause of death, though two patients died of a later cerebral insult.

Therefore thrombotic stroke in the young would seem to represent the normal tail of any frequency distribution, but associated factors of hypertension and diabetes might be more common (see Chapter IX), while non-atherosclerotic disease, whether of congenital, specific arteritic, or other medical nature, would provide most of the cases in children.

Before we look at the clinical subdivisions for the general group of thromboembolic disorders, we might consider briefly some of the anatomic material of pertinence.

Autopsy Data in Thromboembolism. Moossy's investigations in New Orleans (1959—1966) are worthy of careful study. For a time, his seemed the lone voice crying that yes, Virginia, there are intracranial occlusions. He was able to find evidence of intracranial lesions pertinent to infarcts in about half his stroke patients at autopsy [1965, 1966 (2), 1966 (3)]. In an unselected series of 2650 consecutive autopsies 5% of the patients had recent encephalomalacia. The frequency distribution of the lesions by age and sex of the patients is in Appendix Table VII—a—8; median age in each sex was about 63 years. A similar distribution for intracranial occlusions in 4000 autopsies in New York was described by Aronson (1966). Median age for his patients with occlusions was 69, as opposed to 64 years for all autopsies. The frequency of occlusions among autopsies (age-specific rates) rose from 1% at 26 to 35 to 9% at 76 to 85 (Appendix Table VII—a—9). More than 5% of all patients over the age of 45 had intracranial occlusions.

In a smaller series, Moossy (1959) found parenchymal lesions in $^1/_3$ (age 30 to 39) to $^1/_2$ (age 70 and over) of brains examined. Evidence of cerebral arteriosclerosis was present in *all* patients above age 30 at least. "Complicated" arteriosclerosis (hemorrhage, thrombi, and/or calcium in the plaques) was present in 10% of those age 30 to 49 and $^1/_3$ of those age 70 or more (Appendix Table VII—a—10).

The anatomic distribution of thromboembolic occlusions in some 1000 autopsies is described by Jörgensen (1966) at Oslo. Half the occlusions were in the carotid system, equally divided between intracranial and extracranial. An additional $^1/_4$ were in the middle cerebral, and branches or trunks of the posterior circuit comprised the last $^1/_4$. Anterior cerebral occlusions were 3%. Interesting differences were found for recent thrombotic vs. recent embolic occlusions: in the former, $^2/_3$ were in the carotid system, middle cerebral was 7%, and the remainder were in the posterior circulation; intracranial and extracranial carotid involvement was still equal. The emboli, as one might expect, were 60% in the middle cerebral, and 20% in the carotid, almost all intracranial (Appendix Table VII—a—11).

Battacharji (1967) in England pointed out the equal frequency (30%) of severe stenosis of the middle cerebral *and* posterior cerebral arteries, and the marked discrepancy in cerebral infarcts in the territory of each, being of course infrequent with the latter. He showed a modest correlation between the degree of intracranial and extracranial stenosis for patients *without* infarcts, but none for those *with* cerebral lesions. He felt that extracranial stenosis was more severe in the infarct patients than in his controls, but his figures look more discrepant to me for the intracranial vessels. Multiplicity of vascular involvement was the rule.

At the Mayo Clinic, MARTIN (1960) studied the extracranial vessels in 100 consecutive autopsies of patients over age 50. All individuals showed atherosclerotic changes, and at least one artery was totally occluded in 11% (3% who had two vessels occluded and 9 of whom had another severely sclerotic). In all, the occlusion was in the proximal internal carotid; the multiple closures being two in a vertebral and one in a contralateral carotid. An additional 29% had at least one major vessel whose lumen was diminished to less than half its original area. Most patients had *no* neurologic symptoms; $^8/_{14}$ occlusions and $^3/_4$ of stenotic lesions had never produced symptoms of focal or diffuse cerebral involvement.

The "carotid steal" syndrome of reversed blood flow in the posterior circuit has been popular since its first description (REIVICH, 1961). It has been described

Table VII – 2. *Percentage frequency distribution for age of patients with carotid system vs. verte-brobasilar occlusion in three clinical series*

Carotid GURDJIAN (1961)		McDOWELL		Vertebrobasilar McDOWELL	WILLIAMS	
age	%	age	%	%	age	%
35—50	26	< 51	25	12	< 50	20
51—65	58	51—65	30	36	50—59	29
		61—70	30	36	60—69	22
66—76	16	71 ≤	16	16	70 ≤	29
Total	100		101	100		100
N	98		57	50		65
mean age	56		59	62		60*

* Median

too with lesions of the innominate artery (BLAKEMORE, 1965), as a bilateral entity (CODER, 1965), and as a sequel of correcting congenital cardiac defects (FOLGER, 1965). As a numerical part of our current problem, it is extremely minor.

The location of encephalomalacic areas was cerebral in 78% of instances, brain stem in 12%, and cerebellar in 11% in ARONSON's series (1966). Within the cerebrum, relative frequency by lobe was in accord with its size, but 30% involved the basal ganglia alone; this is $^1/_4$ of all infarcts (Appendix Table VII—a—12). The distribution of all infarcts was therefore quite proportional to the volume of grey tissue present with which of course the degree of vascularization is highly correlated. Extensive collaterals would seem to protect the thalamic regions.

Clinical Components of Thromboembolism. The age distribution of thrombosis as a whole has been described above. There is no difference of note in age for lesions of the carotid vs. vertebrobasilar system (Table VII—2). Since one of the authors reached a contrary conclusion, the data were formally tested, and indeed no significant difference could be found (Appendix Table VII—a—13).

Subdivisions of thrombosis-embolism, as listed in Chapter II, were thrombosis (divided into "stroke in evolution" and "completed stroke"), embolism, "thorem", and TIA. Some data on relative frequencies of the components are presented in Table VII–3. The source is FISHER's study (1961) from seven centers in the United States. Since there are no data on non-stroke patients, the male preponde-

Table VII–3. *Percentage frequency distributions by types and locales for cerebral thrombosis-embolism from cooperative stroke study in 7 centers in USA* (FISHER)

Type	M/F ratio	Locale			Total	
		IC	V–B	unknown	N	%
Transient Ischemic Attack	2.56	56.3	37.5	6.3	32	8.4
Thrombosis in Evolution	1.15	55.0	40.0	5.0	100	26.3
(Completed) Thrombosis	3.21	77.1	18.7	4.2	118	31.1
Total Thrombosis	1.93	67.0	28.4	4.6	218	57.4
Thorem	1.43	91.2	7.8	1.0	102	26.8
Embolism	0.93	92.9	7.1	—	28	7.4
Total (N)	1.72	284	84	13	380	—
Total (%)	—	74.7	22.1	3.2	—	100.0

IC = internal carotid system
V–B = vertebrobasilar system
thorem = *th*rombosis *or* *em*bolism

Table VII–4. *Relative frequency of cerebral thrombosis vs. embolism*

Source	Years	Embo-lism	Throm-bosis	Total Ischemic CVD	ratio	ratio
		(A)	(B)	(C)	(A/B)	(A/C)
I — Autopsy data						
Oslo, Norway (JÖRGENSEN)	1959	78	170	320	0.46	0.24
II — Hospital series						
Frederiksberg, Denmark (DALSGAARD)	1940—1953	68	500	568	0.14	0.12
USA, 7 centers (FISHER)	1958—1959	27	217	378*	0.12	0.07*
New York (GROCH)	1956—1960	36	493	539	0.07	0.07
Lake Co., Ill. (ERICSON)	1963	9	100	109	0.09	0.08
Middlesex, Engl. (CARTER)	1952—1961	108	612	720	0.18	0.15
III — Population surveys						
Goulburn, Austral. (WALLACE)	1962—1964	10	101	111	0.10	0.09
Framingham, Mass. (KANNEL)	1949—1962	13	57	70	0.23	0.19
Middlesex, Conn. (EISENBERG)	1957—1958	4	91	95	0.04	0.04

* The additional 102 were classed as "thorem"

rance is difficult to interpret. In general, TIA were 8% of thromboembolic stroke, thrombosis 57% (about half considered "evolving "when seen), thrombosis *or* embolism ("thorem") 27%, and embolism 7%. "Thrombosis in evolution" or "ingravescent stroke" (CARTER, 1960) seems in large measure an artefact of the physician's being present early after the insult, though it is certainly true some strokes progress even over days. In locale, carotid system thromboses were about twice as common as vertebrobasilar. TIA acted like thrombosis. Embolism and "thorem" behaved alike with 9 out of 10 in the carotid tree. On this basis one might surmise that "thorem" is the cautious clinician's embolism and TIA is related to thrombosis. If the former were true, however, embolism would be half as common as thrombosis, which does not meet clinical expections (mine, anyhow).

Table VII–5. *Distribution of TIA by site and sex from several studies*

Sex	Study	Site		
		Carotid	Vertebrobasilar	Total
Male	(1)	52	39	91
	(2)	32	17	49
	(3)	19	9	28
	Total	103	65	168 + 87* = 255
	%	61.3	38.7	100.0 (66.1) (69.3)
Female	(1)	30	37	67
	(2)	3	7	10
	(3)	6	3	9
	Total	39	47	86 + 27* = 113
	%	45.4	54.6	100.0 (33.9) (30.7)
Total	(1)	82	76	158
	(2)	35	24	59
	(3)	25	12	37
	Total	142	112	254 + 114* = 368
	%	55.9	44.1	100.0 (100.0) (100.0)
	*	56	56	112
	(6)	30	30	60
	Σ	228	198	426
	%	53.5	46.5	100.0

(1) MARSHALL; (2) BURROWS; (3) PEARCE; * = [(4) J. ACHESON + (5) FISHER]; (6) BAKER

Accordingly, more information was sought, and, like all Gaul, divided into our three parts, "autopsy data" supplanting "mortality statistics" (Table VII–4). Frequencies are variable, but in general would suggest that only about 10% of thromboembolic occlusive disease is embolism. The higher proportion in JÖRGEN-SEN's autopsy series (1966) is explicable on the basis that common causes of emboli are also common causes of death, unrelated to the cerebrum, or that cerebral embolism more often results in early death than cerebral thrombosis, if we assume this to be a real difference.

Transient Ischemic Attacks. The modern-day equivalent of "cerebral artery spasm" seems to be the less-arbitrary "TIA", which has been ascribed to micro-emboli, sludging, or local ischemia or hypotension, *inter alia*. We saw in FISHER's series about 8% of thromboembolic stroke were so classed. Perhaps the most authoritative account of the disorder is found in JOHN MARSHALL's work [1964 (1)]. In Appendix Table VII—a—14 are distributions by age, sex, and locale for TIA in London. There is little variation in age by either sex or location, the mean being 59 years. Males predominated in the carotid TIA (1.7 ratio), but were equal in the vertebrobasilar.

Table VII—5 contains a condensation of sex and site distribution from this and other major studies. Overall the carotid tree was involved in 54% of TIA,

Table VII–6. *Percentage frequency distributions for various characteristics of Transient Ischemic Attacks (TIA) in London* (MARSHALL)

	Carotid	Vertebro-basilar	Total
A — Frequency			
1 or 2	65	40	52
3-"several"	17	29	23
"many"	18	31	25
Total	100	100	100
N	60	68	128
B — Duration of episodes			
minutes	41	63	52
½ hour	13	11	12
1 hour	12	7	9
several hours	34	20	27
Total	100	100	100
N	68	75	143
C — Duration (onset to admission) for those with more than one TIA			
< 1 month	50	20	30
1—12 months	13	10	11
1—3 years	19	47	37
3—10 years	19	23	22
Total	101	100	100
N	16	30	46

but this apparently differed by sex, being 61% in males and 45% in females. Read percentages horizontally for these frequencies. The sex ratio in TIA as a whole is quite clearly 2 to 1 male to female. Though more discrepant in the carotid TIA, this was still true of the vertebrobasilar (1.38). These percentages are read vertically, on the right-hand side. Just as with the differences by sex we had observed with aneurysms, this too seems to me an inexplicable finding.

One last feature of TIA is worth some attention. MARSHALL [1964 (1)] commented on the greater number of attacks reported in those whose vertebrobasilar tree was involved. The basis for this statement is in the part A of Table VII—6. However, when we look at part C, duration of the illness, the opposite picture emerges, and one would need to know "attacks per patient-month at risk" before any conclusion about frequency versus site would be warranted. As to the duration of the individual episodes, I can see no striking difference between the two sites, though carotid appear longer.

Sex Ratios in Thromboembolism. To finish this segment, we once again look at the male/female ratios in our tripartite resources. Unity was the observation in Danish mortality rate data, but a female preponderance in England (Appendix Table VII—a—15). Hospital series varied. Those containing over 400 cases were 0.84, 0.73, 0.91, and 1.04. Lesser numbers revealed 2.06, 2.22, 1.72; and 3.06 in the smallest (65 cases). These ratios were based on the number of cases, and the highest frequencies of males were in the series of younger-aged patients. The population survey ratios based on cases were 0.8—0.9; using incidence rate ratios they were 1.13 (median age 59) and 0.83 (age 75), but numbers in both are small, being 57 and 91 cases.

Male/female ratios for age-specific mortality rates in Denmark showed a male preponderance in the younger ages (about 1.7 near age 50) falling to unity in the elderly for category 332. In "other" CVD (334), a male excess of about 1.2 or less was present without a clear relation to age. The total mortality rate ratios were 0.96 and 1.01 for the two categories (Appendix Table VII—a—16).

Data for subdivisions of thromboembolism show unity as the ratio in the autopsy series based on cases, but a ratio of 0.9 when they are based on rates per autopsies. Hospital series are all to small for confidence.

Thus there *may* well be a slight male excess for thromboembolic CVD in the younger years, but this would seem to be in the order of 1.3 or so, which is exceedingly minor in relation to differences by age. In TIA however the male does appear to dominate, even if nowhere else.

References

ACHESON, J. 1
ARONSON 18
AURELL 21
BAKER 22—25
BALOW 26
BATTACHARJI 27
BLAKEMORE 35
BRADSHAW 40
BRYANT 42, 43
BURROWS 50
CARTER 53, 54
CODER 58
DALSGAARD 70
DAVIE 72

DU BOULAY 87
EISENBERG 93
ERICSON 97
FELGER 101
FISHER, C. M. 104—106
FOLGER 113
GOLDBERG 125
GROCH 131, 132
GURDJIAN 133—136
HUSNI 159
JÖRGENSEN 165
KANNEL 169, 170
KURLAND 188
LARSSON 197

LINDGREN 201
LOUIS 208
MARSHALL 216—221
MARTIN 223
McDOWELL 231
MOOSSY 253—257
PEARCE 286
REIVICH 302
ROBINSON 307
WALLACE 379
WELLS 382, 383
WILLIAMS 386
ZIELKE 409

CHAPTER VIII

Race and the Japan Story

In every article dealing with CVD and its racial characteristics, the statement is chorused that CVD (especially cerebral hemorrhage) is much more common in the American Negro than in his white peer, and that the frequencies in Japan are massively higher than anywhere else in the world [ACHESON, 1966 (1); BERKSON, 1965; BORHANI, 1965 (2); GOLDBERG, 1962; HOWARD, 1965; KRUEGER, 1967; NICHAMAN, 1962; ROSE, 1962; STAMLER, 1966; STALLONES, 1965, TROMBOLD, 1966]. KURLAND (1967), in citing the same data, does question the validity of the conclusions. Let us see what the evidence may be.

Table VIII–1. *Approximate age-adjusted average annual mortality rates* by race and sex in cases per 100,000 population for types of CVD in Memphis, Tenn., 1959—1961* (KRUEGER)

	330—334 All CVD	330—331 SAH + Cb. H.	332 Cb. Thr.	334 other
Negro female	200	82	50	68
Negro male	180	73	44	66
White male	140	39	55	46
White female	100	32	36	36

* rates estimated from the published figures

CVD in the American Negro. Inferences as to the frequency of CVD in the Negro by the aforementioned authors are based exclusively on mortality statistics. KRUEGER (1967) cited the high mortality rates of CVD among Negroes in the past 40 years in Memphis, Tennessee, after he reassessed their death certificates. Rates fell but slightly with time in Negroes, in contradistinction to those in whites, and the Negro/white ratios were the highest for cerebral hemorrhage (including SAH) and "other and ill-defined" CVD. Cerebral thrombosis death rates were really not too discrepant. In Table VIII–1 we can see the rates as nearly as I could estimate them from the published figures.

NICHAMAN (1962) in similar fashion reviewed death certificates in Charleston, South Carolina, and concluded CVD was five (male) to ten (female) times as common as a cause of death in Negroes as in whites. He essentially excluded the category of "deaths due to unknown and natural causes", which were "almost one-third of the nonwhite deaths" (p. 727) and some 7% of the white deaths. What he did was redistribute these deaths in the same proportions as those for which a definite cause was listed. Further, in his review he changed the original number of CVD deaths from 628 to 814. In addition, deaths from CVD certified by a coroner were 8 in whites and 43 in Negroes. His calculated age and sex specific CVD mortality rates for Negro deaths are some four to eight times as high as the same rates in Chicago or in the United States as a whole, while his white rates were but little different.

The major evidence though derives from national mortality statistics. In GOLDBERG's study (1962) of international comparisons, to which our attention has been repeatedly drawn, the average annual age-adjusted mortality rate for US Negroes in 1951—1958 was 165 per 100,000 against 95 in the whites. Cerebral

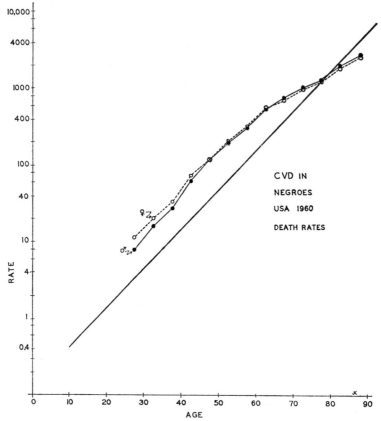

Fig. VIII–1. Age and sex specific annual mortality rates for CVD in non-whites (Negroes) in the United States (1960). Data are in Appendix Table VIII–a–1, from BERKSON (1965)

hemorrhage was 111 vs. 60, thrombosis 28 vs. 23, and ill-defined 20 vs. 9 for Negroes vs. whites. BORHANI [1965 (2)] plotted the national distributions by state for each race and sex, and showed that the Negro CVD deaths were even more concentrated in the southeastern US than the white deaths (see Chapter V). I am confident that the inverse relationship between CVD and physicians in the United States which was drawn in Fig. V–12 for whites would be even stronger for Negroes.

The age and sex specific annual mortality rates for Negro CVD deaths in 1960 are seen in Fig. VIII–1, against our US-England standard of Chapter IV; data

are in Appendix Table VIII—a—1, from BERKSON (1965). Differences between
sexes are minimal but there is no question but that CVD deaths are reported at
least twice as often in Negroes as in whites until we reach the oldest ages. Remember
this is a logarithmic scale, so that doubling the height represents a ten-fold increase.

What support do we have for this being a true reflection of reality ? One
disturbing feature is that in general as we move into the states which might be
presumed better stocked with physicians, the Negro/white discrepancy becomes
much less. In only one of the population surveys we have assessed is there any
direct evidence. PARRISH (1966) in mid-Missouri did find a higher incidence
rate for CVD in Negroes, at 4.1 per 1000 vs. 2.5 in whites. The Negro rate however
was based on but 24 cases, and is further subject to population undercount
discussed below; correction for this would probably bring the Negro rate to less
than 3 per 1000. The Chronic Illness Study of Baltimore (1957) reported *no*
difference in CVD rates between whites and Negroes, but the numbers here too
are too small for confidence. Without citing figures, OSTFELD stated that in his
Old Age Assistance Study in Chicago, "the incidence of new strokes was about
the same in whites and in Negroes" (SIEKERT, 1966, p. 79). He *did* say TIA were
much more frequent in whites; this I would suspect is an ethnic artefact.

CHAPMAN (1966) followed a group of some 1900 male city employees in Los
Angeles for 12 years. In this period there were 36 CVD cases among 1552 whites,
or 2.3% (we need not bother with annual rates). In the same interval there were
4 strokes among 302 Negroes, or 1.3%. While admittedly a small series, certainly
if stroke were excessive in Negroes it should have been somewhat more apparent
in this period.

Other than these bits of information, we have to fall back on hospital series in
our search. In NEFZGER's Cooperative Study (1967) of veterans, 84 or 20% of
CVD patients were Negro. While this would seem far in excess of the 7% of the
veteran population they comprise (House Committee, 1961), it does not *appear*
to me to be a proportion above expectation; utilization of VA hospitals is strongly
influenced by socioeconomic factors. Indeed it is illegal to enter one for treatment
of a non-service-connected illness if the patient can afford other care. As a clinical
impression *only*, I personally have not been struck by any marked excess of stroke
in Negroes in veterans hospitals of New York, Pennsylvania, or Washington, at
which a 20% rate in Negroes would be considered indeed to be low.

HEYMAN (1961) had 47 whites and 21 Negroes among his North Carolina
patients, predominantly at a VA Hospital in this heavily Negro state. LOUIS
(1966) stated the proportion of young stroke patients who were white, Negro,
or Puerto Rican at Bellevue was for each the same as expected from the remainder
of the hospital patients. The only other evidence I could find to this point was
from MEYER (1959) in Detroit, where Negroes comprised 62.7% of his CVD cases —
and 60.3% of all neurologic admissions.

Differences for CVD in other racial groups of the United States have also been
put forth. In Table VIII—2 are age and sex specific rates for CVD deaths in 1950
(BERKSON, 1965). The rates in Negroes have been covered already. Those in the
American Indian are equal to the white. While both oriental rates would *seem* to
be higher, consideration of the total populations listed on the right would indicate
that all age 45 to 54 rates are based on less than 10 cases each, and numbers in the

next decade would not be much greater. Therefore I do not believe this provides evidence of racial differences for Americans of Oriental extraction.

The data available do not indicate to me substantial support either for the mortality-based high frequency of CVD in Negroes. I am inclined to conclude the opposite, that what information there is suggests there is *no* major racial predilection for stroke in the US Negro. The safest statement is that an increased

Table VIII–2. *Age-specific cerebrovascular disease mortality rates in cases per 100,000 in 1950 for US inhabitants by race* (BERKSON)

Race	Age 45—54		Age 55—64		Total pop. (m) (all ages)*	
	M	F	M	F	M	F
Whites	55	55	186	157	67,129.0	67,813.0
Negroes	213	249	523	571	7,298.7	7,743.6
Am. Indians	69	65	182	153	178.8	164.6
Chinese Am.	96	118	349	269	77.0	40.6
Japanese Am.	55	106	230	200	76.6	65.1

* (Statistical History of the United States) 74,833.0   75,864.0

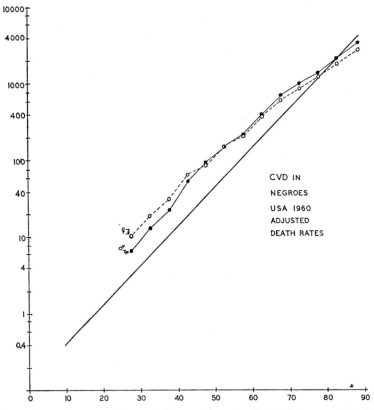

Fig. VIII–2. Age and sex specific annual mortality rates for CVD in non-whites (Negroes) in the United States (1960), as in Fig. VIII—1, but corrected for population bias. Data are in Appendix Table VIII–a–2

frequency in the Negro has not been demonstrated. Earlier comments concerning the uncertainties in cerebral hemorrhage vs. thrombosis from mortality statistics are even more pertinent for the Negro who, as a group, is less under medical supervision than the white. Further there is uniformly an excess in Cb hemorrhage and "other" CVD, and no real difference in thrombosis even in the mortality data. We have seen that "hemorrhage" in the US is incorrectly used for non-specific CVD. Therefore both excesses would appear to be in poorly-defined conditions called stroke, which lends even less credence to the findings. This usage by the way may explain the difference in hemorrhage proportions between the US and England.

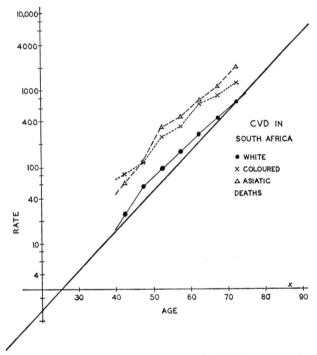

Fig. VIII–3. Age specific average annual mortality rates for CVD by race in those age 40—74 in South Africa (1954—1958). Heavy solid line refers to US-England CVD deaths. Data are in Appendix Table VIII–a–3, from WALKER (1963)

There is yet one more factor to be considered in regard to the Negro stroke deaths, and that is uncertainty as to the denominator. Errors in population enumeration from the decennial census was the general topic of the October 25, 1967 meeting of the Washington Statistical Society, at which JOSEPH WAKSBERG of the Bureau of the Census estimated some 5 million US citizens were missed at the 1960 census. MONROE G. SIRKEN of the National Center for Health Statistics then pointed out the marked variations in undercount by sex, race, and region, and presented an approximation of the degree of bias present in mortality statistics as a result of both population undercounts and age misreporting at death. While in whites the maximum mortality rate error at any age was 5%, in Negroes the deviation was as high as 46%, but with large differences among the age-groups and between the sexes. In Appendix Table VIII—a—2 I have summarized his estimates of the net bias and then recalculated with these corrections the Negro CVD mortality rates from Table VIII—a—1. We can see that most rates are now considerably closer to those of the US whites, with a reduction in the middle ages and an increase in the elderly. However there is still a clear excess, and the data when plotted (Fig. VIII—2) give a curve similar to that of Fig. VIII—1, except that there is no longer the relative decline in those 75 and older.

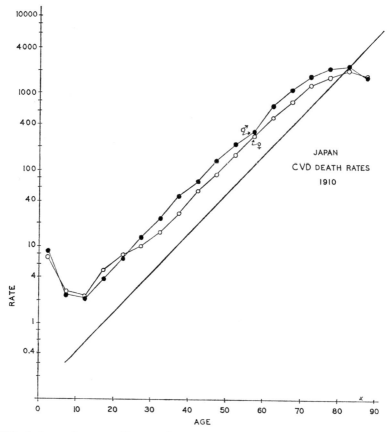

Fig. VIII—4. Age and sex specific annual mortality rate for CVD in Japan (1910). Data are in Appendix Table VIII—a—5

CVD in South Africa. WALKER (1963) published a study on stroke and heart disease in South Africa. For the country as a whole, the average annual age-specific mortality rates for CVD in 1954—1958 are presented in Fig. VIII—3, again against the US-England standard. That for whites is essentially the same as our criterion. The Coloured (mixed) and Asiatic (Indian) mortality rates would seem much higher, but the total population on which the rates are based was but 1.5 million in the former and 500,000 in the latter (Appendix Tables VIII—a—3). These rates look very similar to those of the US Negro. I have no direct information on the availability of medical facilities to these racial groups in South Africa.

WALKER also presented his data from CVD deaths in hospital in Johannesburg, South Africa among the same races and the Bantu (Appendix Table VIII–a–4). Numbers are small in all groups, and I do not discern any real difference by age or sex in the proportion of CVD to total deaths between the whites and the Bantu. With even smaller numbers, rates would *seem* somewhat higher in Coloured and Asiatic. As an approximation, for those age 65 and over some 6% of whites, 7% of Bantu, 10% of Coloured, and 12% of Asiatic deaths were so classed. I would believe the topic warrants further study, but at present a racial predilection in South Africa would also appear unproven.

CVD in Japan. The most weight in the racial story has been given to the phenomenal frequencies reported for CVD in Japan. In GOLDBERG's international comparison, the age-adjusted mortality rate was 209 per 100,000 (vs. 100 per

Table VIII–3. *Causes of death in Japan 1900—1960 (cases per 100,000 pop.)* *

Year	Pop. (millions)	CVD	Malignant Neoplasms	Heart Disease	Life Expectancy M	F
1900	43.8	159	46	48	44	45
1905	46.6	163	57	55		
1910	49.2	132	67	65	44	45
1915	52.8	129	72	64		
1920	56.0	158	73	64	42	43
1925	59.7	161	71	67		
1930	64.5	163	71	64	45	47
1935	69.3	165	72	58	47	50
1940	71.9	178	72	63	(24)	(38) ← 1943
1947	78.1	129	69	62	50	54
1950	83.2	127	77	64	58	62
1955	89.3	136	87	61	64	68
1960	93.4	161	100	73	65	70

* crude rates

100,000 for the mean of 18 countries). The rate for cerebral hemorrhage alone was 180. That this has been a situation of long standing is indicated in Table VIII–3, where the crude (unadjusted) death rates for CVD are seen to have been generally about 150 per 100,000 through the entirety of this century. Carcinoma and heart disease rates have increased *pari passu* with life expectancy (Ministry of Health and Welfare, 1962).

The age-specific annual mortality rates for CVD by sex in Japan in 1910 are presented in Fig. VIII–4, against the US-England experience (Appendix Table VIII–a–5). The marked excess up to the oldest ages is obvious. A male preponderance is also very clear.

Similar are the findings for 1950 (Fig. VIII–5) and for 1962 (Fig. VIII–6), with data in Appendix Table VIII–a–12. Populations are listed in Appendix Table VIII–a–6, and the succeeding tables a–7 through a–12 contain the age and sex specific rates for the subdivisions of CVD (330 to 334) in 1950 and 1962.

In contrast to 1910, the CVD death rates of 1950 are notably closer to our standard, especially at the younger ages, and sex differences are far less obvious.

By 1962, the younger rates have reached the base, but once again there appears a notable excess in males, and rates are still much higher than in US-England for most of the range.

As we can see in Table VIII—4, the proportion of deaths in the elderly provided by CVD deaths are at present twice as high as contemporaneous experience elsewhere (see Chapter IV). Even 50 years ago, with "degenerative" diseases forming a much smaller fraction of deaths, the percentage was high.

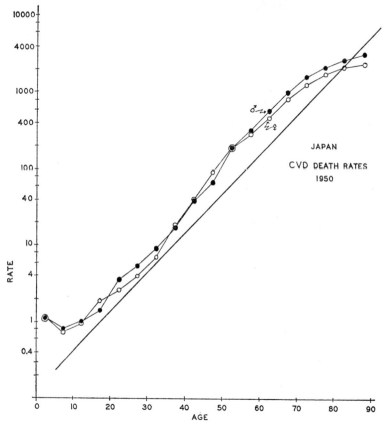

Fig. VIII—5. Age and sex specific annual mortality rate for CVD in Japan (1950). Data are in Appendix Tables VIII—a—12

In terms of the type of CVD, in 1950 92% of all CVD deaths were classed as cerebral hemorrhage (331). By 1962 they comprised 71%, and we have estimated elsewhere from western experience they should be some 30% of CVD deaths. SAH was 2 (1950) to 4 (1962) cases per 100,000, comparable to occidental rates. Cerebral thrombosis-embolism rose from 4 to 28 per 100,000 in this interval, and "other and ill-defined" *also* rose, from 3 to 16 per 100,000 (Appendix Table VIII—a—7 thru 11).

TAKAHASHI (1957, 1961) indicated that CVD deaths were concentrated in the northern part of the main island of Japan; major population and university centers superficially appeared to me to be low frequency areas.

Data similar to that already presented for Japan and the Japanese Americans were used by GORDON (1957) to show that Hawaiian Japanese CVD death rates were intermediate between the two. The Hawaiian age and sex specific rates were based on less than 400 cases in three years from my reconstruction, and really looked quite similar to US rates. The Hawaiian rates rose from about 17 per 100,000 at age 35 to 44 to some 600 at age 65 to 74. Comparable US *white* rates are 13 and some 500. BENNETT (1962) found the Japanese Hawaiian CVD death rates

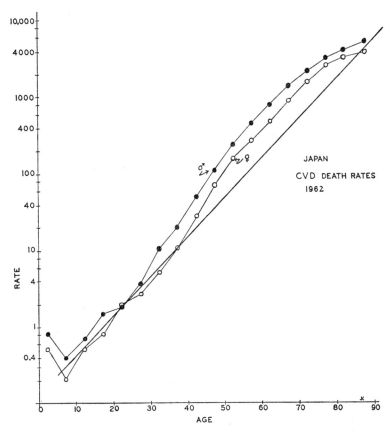

Fig. VIII—6. Age and sex specific annual mortality rates for CVD in Japan (1962). Data are in Appendix Table VIII—a—12

at 160 per 100,000 age 35 to 74 were identical to those of the other islanders combined. He claimed the Polynesians had the highest rates (240) and the Hawaiian whites the lowest (110). Numbers of CVD deaths in the last two groups are about 300 and 400 each. Small numbers give small reliability; this, with the racial admixture of Hawaii, would make conclusions from mortality data especially uncertain here.

The Dénouement. A population sample of some 22,000 adults living in 18 areas of Japan was described by BERKSON (1965) in support of a high rate of CVD in that land (Table VIII—5). KATSUKI [1964 (2)] provides further details on that study, of which his Hisayama project is one part. Fourteen university centers were responsible for conducting the study.

Note (Table VIII—5) that CVD was considered the cause in 36% of all deaths in those age 40 or more in this study. Cerebral hemorrhage was somewhat over

Table VIII—4. *Proportions of CVD deaths to all deaths in Japan by sex for those aged 60 or over*

		Male	Female	Total
1910	age 60 ≤			
	CVD	23,714	20,936	44,650
	all deaths	136,300	137,100	273,400
	%	17.40	15.27	16.33
1910	age 65 ≤			
	CVD	18,242	17,059	35,301
	all deaths	103,900	112,600	216,500
	%	17.56	15.15	16.31
1962	age 60 ≤			
	CVD	67,464	63,351	130,815
	all deaths	232,345	224,085	456,430
	%	29.04	28.27	28.66
1962	age 65 ≤			
	CVD	55,300	55,873	111,173
	all deaths	192,534	199,779	392,313
	%	28.72	27.97	28.34

Table VIII—5. *Deaths in 1962—1963 among Japanese "population sample" of 21800 aged 40 or more (from Okinaka, cited by* BERKSON)

ISC	Cause	No.	Annual rate*	% of deaths	% CVD
330	SAH	5	23	1.1	3.1
331	Cb. H.	92	422	20.1	56.4
332	Cb. thr.	44	202	9.6	27.0
334	CVD, other	22	101	4.8	13.5
330—334	CVD	163	748	35.6	100.0
	Heart disease	62	284	13.5	38.0

    * cases per 100,000 population age *40 or more*

half the CVD — a considerable change from the national figures seen in Japan above in this chapter.

Of the 163 CVD deaths, 21 or 13% were autopsied [KATSUKI, 1964 (2)].

In this and other papers, KATSUKI (1964, 1966) described the changing proportions in cerebral hemorrhage/thrombosis deaths in Japan from 29 to 1 in 1951 to 4 to 1 in 1962. He attributes this dramatic alteration largely to an increase in thrombosis.

The final act of our drama consists of a detailed look at the important survey of KATSUKI in Hisayama, Japan (1964, 1966).

Hisayama is a rural community at the outskirts of Fukuoka on Kyushu Island, ten miles from Kyushu University. Population was some 6800 in 1958—1961.

KATSUKI has followed carefully all adults age 40 and over in Hisayama since 1961. He has tabulated the number and type of CVD deaths for the four years from November, 1961. In Table VIII—6 are listed his results, incorporating his most recent material [KATSUKI, 1966 (1), (2)]. Several features stand out:

1. Autopsy rates for year 1 were 15%, and soon became virtually complete

Table VIII—6. *Final diagnoses for CVD cases in Hisayama, Japan, in population survey of 1600 inhabitants over age 40, from* KATSUKI *[1966 (1, 2)], between 1961 and 1965*

Type	Year 1			Year 2			Year 3 + 4			Total		
	N	d.	(*)	N	d.	(*)	N	d.	(*)	N	d.	(*)
Cb. H.	7	6	(3)	2	2	(2)	4	3	(3)	13	11	(8)
Cb. thr.	6	2	(1)	7	3	(3)	19	7	(7)	32	12	(11)
Cb. Emb.	1	1	(1)	0	—		0	—	—	1	1	(1)
SAH	1	1	(1)	1	1	(1)	1	1	(1)	3	3	(3)
Other	3	3	(0)	0	—		0	—	—	3	3	(0)
Total	18	13	(6)	10	6	(6)	24	11	(11)	52	30	(23)
(1) Total autopsies	6			18			65			89		
(2) Total deaths	41			20			66			127		
(3) % (1)/(2)	15%			90%			99%			70%		

* = number autopsied
d. = number of deaths
N = number of cases

2. CVD deaths comprised 32% of total deaths in year 1 and 17% in years 3 and 4.

3. Cerebral hemorrhage/thrombosis deaths in year 1 were 6/2; in years 3 and 4, they were 3/7.

The results are actually even more dramatic than cited here, since the final diagnostic revisions of the material have been cited. In Appendix Table VIII—a—13 are the findings as originally reported [KATSUKI, 1964 (1), (2)]: in the first year and a half there were then considered to be 10 hemorrhage and 3 thrombosis deaths.

In other words, with autopsy control, CVD in Hisayama has approximated western experience in its frequency as a cause of death and in the hemorrhage/thrombosis ratios.

Another study from Japan is pertinent. The Atomic Bomb Casualty Commission and the Japanese National Institute of Health have been following carefully the survivors of Hiroshima and Nagasaki. From this source, JOHNSON (1967) has reported on CVD in Hiroshima. Between 1958—1964 there were 132 "definite" cases of CVD, which can be summarized as follows:

ISC	CVD cases	Death, CVD		Death, other		Death, Σ	
330	8	7	(7)	0	—	7	(7)
331	30	19	(15)	3	(2)	22	(17)
332	75	12	(9)	47	(45)	59	(54)*
334	19	2	(—)	2	(—)	4	(—)
total	132	40	(31)	52	(47)	92	(78)

No. of autopsies in parentheses
* 34/54 had old cerebral infarcts

There were an additional 43 "unsubstantiated" CVD of which most had been classed as cerebral hemorrhage. Of the 175 total, 87 were male and 88 female. The figures cited are much better than the unselected material would indicate. JOHNSON said that in only 22 % of deaths attributed to CVD was there autopsy confirmation that some type of CVD was directly related to death. Almost $1/_3$ of fatal cerebral thrombosis had been called cerebral hemorrhage.

The ratio in this study *with autopsy control* was 0.4 hemorrhage to thrombosis.

JABLON (1966) provides the *coup de grâce*, I believe. Again from the ABCC study, there were through 1962, 1215 autopsies in Hiroshima and Nagasaki; 675 in 1961—1962, and the remainder in 1950—1960. Autopsy rate for CVD deaths 1950—1960 was 3.2%; it was 25% in the next year, and 43% in the last year — all similar to total autopsy rates per period. Of the 201 autopsied cases classed as any type of CVD (330—334), *only 20 or 10% were confirmed at autopsy*, and an additional 14 were first discovered this way.

In other words, I believe the evidence is good that a high frequency of cerebral hemorrhage — and probably of all CVD — in Japan is nothing more than an artefact of diagnostic fashion, and that there is no evidence here either that there is a racial predilection for CVD.

References

ACHESON, R. M. 5
BENNETT 29
BERKSON 30
BORHANI 37
Bureau de la Statistique Générale 45—47
CHAPMAN 56
Commission on Chronic Illness 60
DALAL 69
Division of Health and Welfare Statistics 81
ERICSON 97
GOLDBERG 125

GORDON, T. 129
Health and Welfare Statistics Division 146
HEYMAN 148—150
House Committee 155
HOWARD, J. 157
JABLON 161
JOHNSON 164
KATSUKI 172—176
KOJIMA 182
KRUEGER 185
KURLAND 188
MEYER 242

Ministry of Health and Welfare 251
NEFZGER 267
NICHAMAN 269
PARRISH 283
ROSE 309, 310
SIEKERT 325
SIRKEN 327
STAMLER 335
STALLONES 336
TAKAHASHI 355, 356
TROMBOLD 365
WAKSBERG 377
WALKER 378

Chapter IX

Factors Associated with CVD

We have considered already the equivocal relationship between the occurrence of CVD and sex or race. The very striking effects of age upon its frequency (except for SAH) have also been noted, and stroke in young adults would best seem to represent the tail expected in any frequency distribution. We might now inquire into those factors which have been claimed to be causative or precipitating in CVD. This necessarily entails speaking to the point of the associated disorders themselves, at least in sketchy outline. Only disorders recently considered related entities will be under review. Older claims, such as an inverse relationship of CVD and CA, especially in women, seem not to have attracted the interest of current workers.

The major features associated with SAH have been mentioned previously (and see Giel, 1965), while the common causes for cerebral embolism (see Wells, 1959) are for the most part the obvious cardiac ills producing mural thrombi and arhythmia.

Hypertension. In our general experience we ordinarily expect a rise with age in blood pressure levels, especially the systolic. The British Medical Journal commented editorially (1967) on the importance of a new concept, that rise in blood pressure with age is chiefly a function of the pressure levels themselves rather than a consequence of age. This concept arose from the study of Miall (1967) on blood pressure levels over some ten years in South Wales from longitudinal population surveys. While a trend of increasing pressure with age was present, he claimed with multiple regression analysis that the changes with time were chiefly the result of the mean blood pressure levels: individuals with high mean pressures show a greater degree of change with time than those with low. Mean blood pressure was defined as the average (separately for systolic and diastolic) between the reading at the start of the study and that at the end. He used this measurement because "if the change is related to the mean of the two measurements; these are independent variables" (p. 661). If a is the original reading and b the final, he properly points out that change = (b−a) is not independent of the original reading if one used (b−a)/a. But I fail to see how (b−a)/(b+a) ½ is any less so. Both seem likely to run the risk of "spurious correlation" (Yule, 1950, p. 330). It is possible that it is precisely this spurious correlation that his regression analysis identifies, and therefore that his basic thesis is fallacious. Take two patients (or 200) with identical initial pressures of 100 and with final pressures of 120 and of 200 each. The ratios of Miall are 20/110 and 100/150, and therefore "changes in pressure . . . are highly significantly related to mean pressures", and "the higher the pressure, the greater the rate of increase" (p. 664). Of more import though, in each group by age, sex, or locale, almost all the changes he depicts were positive. In other words, regardless of these factors *or* original pressure levels (or regression coefficients), final pressures were most often higher than those some 10 years earlier.

THORNER (1962) however was unable to find any evidence of change in blood pressure with time in a 6-year cohort study, though at the start of the study there was a very *slight* gradient of pressure with age. As he states this time interval is too short to settle the age-blood pressure question.

The epidemiology of hypertension has been reviewed by, *inter alia*, GEIGER (1963), whose major conclusion seemed to be that the available data on the disorder(s) were inadequate for firm statements, except for the reasonably consistent evidence of a high rate of hypertension in the American Negro. PAUL (1965) writes that "hypertension is concentrated in the obese, the Negro, the middle-aged and elderly, and among those with a lineage of hypertension ... It is likely that the prevalence of hypertension is decreasing in the United States, but the reasons for the decrease are unclear" (p. 114). PAFFENBARGER [1966 (1)] in Memphis described a marked decrease in hypertensive death rates (ISC 440—447) over the previous 20 years for whites but with little change in the much higher Negro rate. JAN HOWARD (1965) called attention to a similar trend from national mortality statistics, and thought this could best be explained by effective treatment of hypertension in whites vs. Negroes, an opinion properly disputed by PAUL (1965). The excess of Negro deaths is mostly in those under age 65 [ROSE, 1962 (1)]. KRUEGER [1966 (2)] has demonstrated a definite decline in hypertensive deaths among US veterans age 55 to 74; rates in 1954 to 1957 were 122 per 100,000 as underlying and 189 as associated cause of death; in 1961 to 1962 these rates were 63 and 115. The validity of decreasing hypertensive deaths, while not in our province here, should be considered with the questions raised in Chapter XI where we look at the problems concerning a decrease in cerebral hemorrhage death reports.

Hypertensive deaths are generally concentrated in the eastern half of the U.S. between New York and the Carolinas; the pattern for Negroes is similar but more concentrated in the southern part of this region [ROSE, 1962 (2)]. That author thought this might be related to population density. In other races SCHROEDER (1958) disputed the general opinion that hypertension was rare in the Orient, outside of Japan, with data mostly based on hospital records. TAKAHASHI (1961, 1957) cited rather impressive rates of hypertension in Japan: at least half the farmers over age 30 he examined had pressures above 150/90.

Effective treatment of malignant hypertension will prolong life and reduce the frequency of its major complications, which are cerebral vascular, cardiac, and renal diseases in roughly equal proportions. Support for this affirmation may be found in the references cited. Less certain are the results in reference to CVD of treating less severely elevated pressures. Hypertensive encephalopathy is well reviewed by JELLINEK (1964).

The relationships of CVD, coronary artery disease (CAD), and hypertension from the geographic distribution of deaths ascribed thereto in Ireland were studied by ACHESON (1960). Correlations were strong in males between CAD and hypertension, and CAD and CVD. Female CAD-CVD and CVD-hypertension rates were not associated, and the remaining permutations seemed moderately related. With the same method though he found that, from standardized mortality rates among 16 countries, only the CAD-hypertension relationships persisted. For CVD and hypertension the correlation coefficients were nearly 0, and for CAD-CVD they were moderately negative within either sex.

Hypertension was present in 31% of non-hemorrhagic stroke patients in one hospital series (MEYER, 1959), and in 51% of another (McDOWELL, 1961). STAMLER (1966) pointed out a progressively increasing risk of CVD with blood pressure levels in men from the data of the Build and Blood Pressure Study of the Society of Actuaries. There were four times as many stroke deaths in men with blood pressures of 148 to 177 systolic over 93 to 102 diastolic than in those with (138 to 147)/ (48 to 82). In the Framingham study KANNEL (1965) found a strong correlation between initial blood pressure levels and later CVD. KURLAND (1967) indicated $2/3$ of CVD patients, regardless of type, were hypertensive according to Mayo Clinic standards.

Insofar as course after stroke, neither ADAMS (1961), BALOW (1967), nor MERRETT (1966) found any relationship between blood pressure and late survival after the ictus.

One strong caution is in order here. From the Baltimore Chronic Illness Study, 21% of the population age 35 to 64, and *41%* 65 or older had hypertension (with or without heart disease). If these rates are valid, almost half the stroke patients would be expected to be hypertensive even if the conditions were totally unrelated.

While hypertension in cerebral hemorrhage is usually considered universally present, rates reported are as low as $2/3$. AURELL (1964) asserted that the decline in cerebral hemorrhage deaths in Göteborg, Sweden was a result of antihypertensive therapy. While the decline is actually not statistically significant (see Chapter X) his statement for the specific patients referred to is worthy of note: none of those under age 65 who had recently died of cerebral hemorrhage had had adequate antihypertensive therapy.

Coronary Artery Disease (CAD) and Arteriosclerosis (AS). That arteriosclerosis is the basic factor underlying non-hemorrhagic stroke is obvious. The question of other sequelae of this pathologic process must therefore be considered. BIÖRCK (1962) of Stockholm declared that case-fatality rates for myocardial infarction rose steadily with age; the peak frequency for CAD deaths in Sweden was in the 70 to 79 decade which is notably higher than in the U.S. From 1935, the mean age had risen to about 70 for female and 65 for male patients with myocardial infarction in 1960, probably a reflection of the rising age-distribution of the population.

ACHESON (1962) thought that on epidemiologic grounds CAD was more a function of "deranged fat metabolism" in the young, while arteriosclerosis was the prime cause in the elderly. Geographic distributions show that CAD deaths in the United States are concentrated on either coast and bear no relation to CVD deaths (BORHANI, 1965; HECHTER, 1965). The latter author reported a random distribution of CAD deaths in California. We have noted ACHESON's Irish study immediately above.

The classic population survey for CAD is the Framingham study (DAWBER, 1959, 1962; KANNEL, 1961). Risk of CAD was directly related to serum cholesterol levels, blood pressure, obesity, cigarette smoking, EKG evidence of left ventricular hypertrophy, diabetes, and diminished vital capacity. Hypertension, EKG changes and smoking but not overweight were similarly related to CAD deaths in BORHANI's study (1963) of longshoremen, though all four factors were present in a similar work (PELL, 1963). SKYRING (1963) found no evidence for an association with smoking or with a number of socioeconomic features. All factors cited though were present in PAFFENBARGER's survey [1966 (2, 3)] of former college students. Prevalence of CAD in Hiroshima, Japan for those age 30 to 59 was $^1/_3$ to $^1/_4$ of the rate in the Framingham study, according to YANO (1963), though the same risk factors including diabetes and obesity were observed. Interestingly, the prevalence of hypertension was the same in both surveys. Similar frequencies and factors for CAD in Japan are recorded in other papers [KATSUKI, 1964 (1), UEDA, 1964, YOSHITOSHI, 1964). In India, NAIK (1966) found little difference between the rates of hospital admissions for CAD and CVD; hypertension was present in half the cases in either category, with diabetes in 4 and 3%. WALKER (1963) in South Africa stated that CAD mortality rates for whites and Indians were at least as high as in England and the U.S., while those for the Coloured were lower. Hospital deaths in Johannesburg were of similar relative magnitudes by race, but Bantu rates here were exceedingly low. WALKER too stressed the differences between CAD and CVD, including the correlations with serum lipids: + for CAD, 0 for CVD.

Since CAD is generally seen at younger ages than CVD, it is not surprising that seldom do CAD studies indicate prior strokes. To the converse, KANNEL (1965) stated that $^3/_4$ of his Framingham stroke patients had prior evidence of cardiovascular disease — mostly hypertension from his later data (1966). STAMLER (1966) cites an increased CVD risk for those with a history of heart disease. In Rochester, KURLAND (1967) found $^1/_3$ of CVD patients had previously some evidence of CAD. Hospital series indicate prior (or coexistent) CAD in varying frequencies.

In the Chronic Illness Study (1957) of Baltimore, the crude prevalence rate for CAD was 23 per 1000 population, hypertensive heart disease 50 per 1000, other non-rheumatic heart disease 16, and hypertension 66 per 1000. Thus 15% of the population had some form of cardiovascular disease, not counting CVD or varicose veins. The rates for the cited categories of course rose strikingly with age. Diabetics accounted for 27 per 1000 population and the CVD rate was 15 per 1000. On this basis, as a rough approximation some 20% of CVD patients would be expected to have prior cardiovascular disease if the entities were totally unrelated. Also, since both CAD and CVD are sequelae of arteriosclerosis and are interrelated too with hypertension and probably diabetes, one would certainly expect to find a high frequency of any of these in CVD. Epidemiologically, CAD and CVD have different age patterns, geographic distributions, sex-ratios, and possibly racial predilections.

The pattern of arteriosclerosis among aorta, coronary, and cerebral arteries is one of progressive increase with age; but in the order cited, there is about a 10-year difference separating each of these three (HOLMAN, 1961).

I would conclude therefore that CAD and CVD are different disorders which are often co-incidental.

Serum Cholesterol and Lipids. In a recent review, McGANDY (1967) believed that lowering the intake of saturated fatty acids and cholesterol will lower their serum levels in humans, which in turn *might* have an effect on the production of atherosclerosis. Though the latter will not be covered here, we should note the strong linear correlation described by CONNOR (1961) between dietary cholesterol and age-adjusted mortality rates for ASHD in 24 countries.

In relation to CVD, MEYER (1959) found a significant elevation of mean cholesterol levels among stroke patients with SAH, aneurysm, hypertension or arteritis, but *not* among those with atherosclerotic CVD. Serum lipid levels showed a similar difference when contrasted with "normals", but no notable variation from other hospitalized patients.

HEYMAN's study (1961) indicated a significant difference between veterans with cerebral infarction and other hospitalized males for serum cholesterol: means were 223 mg-% for 47 white and 235 mg-% for 21 Negro stroke patients vs. 206 and 200 mg-% for the comparison groups. The latter were selected with the expectation they would have "normal" cholesterols. In the stroke patients, the cholesterol level was unaltered by the presence of hypertension and/or ASHD.

ROBINSON (1963) compared 250 patients with cerebral thrombosis with 124 healthy volunteers, and found insignificant elevations of serum cholesterol among the patients. The beta-lipoprotein cholesterol concentrations and the beta/alpha ratios were increased, and usually significantly. Phospholipids were equal. Females with strokes tended to have higher levels of cholesterol. There was some evidence that the elevated lipids were more common in those who died within two years than in the survivors.

KATSUKI [1964 (3)] in Japan found significant elevations only for triglycerides among 31 cerebral infarct patients, though cholesterol and phospholipids also tended to be higher than in controls.

Elevated serum triglycerides were a feature in CVD, according to FELDMAN (1964), among 37 patients with cerebral thrombosis and 26 with cerebrovascular insufficiency. Cholesterol levels were also generally elevated, but most often in association with the triglycerides. The elevations were considerably less common in the CVD patients than in another series with CAD, and were really not markedly different from those of normals aged 40 to 69. Other components of lipid analysis were essentially the same in patients and controls.

In a cooperative study of some 800 veterans, NEFZGER (1967) found that the mean level of serum cholesterol was the same in those with recent cerebral infarct (238 mg-%) as with myocardial infarct (241 mg-%). Though controls were lacking these values would not appear markedly elevated, and are about the same as CUMINGS (1967) reported in his study. The latter could demonstrate no difference for 47 patients who had had a stroke more than 2 years previously vs. 11 controls; tested were triglycerides, cholesterol free and total, phospholipids, and fractionated fatty acids.

Therefore it may be concluded that the evidence linking any of these varied lipid components with cerebral vascular disease is as yet inadequate to establish such a relationship. KANNEL (1966) did feel that an elevated cholesterol before age 50 was a useful *predictor* of later stroke; this needs confirmation; his data (1965) are suggestive only (P < 0.05) by trend analysis of three groups.

Smoking. The relationship between cigarette smoking and bronchogenic carcinoma needs no repetition, and that with smoking and heart disease seems well established. What is the evidence with strokes? In CROFTON's study (1963) in England, Wales, and Scotland there was *no* apparent relationship with smoking, since there was no change in the male/female ratio for CVD deaths among 10-year cohorts born between 1846 and 1915; with this method definite changes were found for bronchogenic CA, pulmonary TB, bronchitis, probably ischemic heart disease, and possibly peptic ulcer. KANNEL (1965) though found an increased risk of CVD among smokers.

Three other prospective studies of importance do give us more direct information. DOLL (1966) provided the results for almost 5000 deaths among British physicians in relation to smoking habits, and classed CVD as an "unrelated cause". However, from his Appendix Table 1, the average mortality rate for CVD was 0.8 per 1000 among non-smokers and 1.5 among smokers, or a ratio of 1.9 to 1.0 if we set the non-smokers at unity. Cigarettes here seemed less discrepant than pipe or cigar smokers, and ex-smokers seemed to have a higher rate than those who continued.

HAMMOND (1964, 1966) has followed one million U.S. citizens since 1960. There is a moderate excess of CVD deaths among smokers. If the mortality ratio for non-smokers is set at 1.0 the ratio for male smokers is 1.5 to 1.4 between age 45 and 74, and for females 2.1 to 1.4. The 75 to 84 decade ratios were 0.9 male and 1.2 female.

KAHN (1966) published the DORN study of U.S. World War I veterans. Again if we set the non-smoker ratio at 1.00, the CVD mortality ratios for current cigarette smokers were 1.40, 1.07 for ex-smokers, and 1.06 for pipe-cigar users. Among the cigarette smokers, the under-10-a-day-cigarettes ratio was 1.26, 10 to 20 was 1.33, 21 to 39 was 1.54, and 40 + was 1.88.

Other Associated Factors. The frequency of diabetes in thrombotic CVD would seem in the order of 13% (MEYER, 1959) to 16% (McDOWELL, 1961), though some series are notably lower, such as GURDJIAN's (1961) rate of 6%. KURLAND's work (1967) indicated 15% were diabetic. About 5% of the population above age 34 were diabetic in the Chronic Diseases Study of Baltimore (1957). Interrelationships of diabetes and hypertension (PELL, 1967) are also pertinent to its specificity in CVD. A moderate increase in CVD mortality with increasing weight was cited by STAMLER (1966) from the Society of Actuaries study, more obvious in men; no such trend was found by KANNEL (1965).

Familial features in CVD have received little attention. HARVALD (1965) has been conducting a study of all twins born in Denmark between 1870—1910, of whom some 6900 pairs have been evaluated. The monozygotic twins (MZ) number 1528 and the same-sexed dizygotic (DZ_1), 2609. In this study, the concordance rates for cardiovascular disease are as follows:

Disease	MZ	DZ_1 (same sex)	DZ_2 (opposite sex)
CAD	20/102	24/155	10/133
Hypertension	20/80	10/106	4/106
CVD	22/98	16/148	22/179

This means that of 122 MZ twins with CAD, the other MZ twin had this diagnosis in 20 instances. It may therefore be seen that the CAD rates (coronary occlusion) do not differ significantly between MZ and DZ twins, and therefore this study provides no evidence for genetic effects. Hypertension *is* significantly greater

(P < 0.01) in MZ, and stroke may also be of import (P < 0.05), compatible with the thesis that genetic factors do play a role in these two disorders.

GIFFORD (1966) said that the parents of 126 stroke patients were reported to have died of cerebrovascular disease at a frequency more than four times expectation (28 mothers and 20 fathers vs. 6.0 and 6.7 expected), though siblings differed little. Heart disease and deaths from all causes showed O/E ratios only slightly above unity. The cause of death was determined from the original death certificate.

The possibility that oral contraceptives are related to the risk of stroke has of course been considered. ILLIS (1965) was unable to find any correlation with their use among angiographically-proven CVD at the National Hospital, and a similarly reassuring result was reported by JENNETT (1967) in Glasgow. However, BICKERSTAFF (1967) did claim an association. While he had been accustomed to seeing but two or three women with cerebral insufficiency annually among those under 45, in the three years to 1966 he encountered 25, of whom 18 had been taking "the pill" with all but five under age 35. SHAFEY (1966) and COLE (1967) each reported on six strokes with the pill. Considering though the first two studies and the many women at risk, one should I believe have had by now more evidence were there any notable association.

DINGWALL-FORDYCE (1963) has called attention to an excess of deaths attributed to CVD in a follow-up of former lead workers. The study was designed to evaluate an increased risk of carcinoma in this group (which was not found). Men were classed by the degree of exposure; Grade C includes those with urinary lead excretion in excess of 100 µg/l. Deaths exceeded expectation only for those in Grade C. Nineteen of the 80 deaths in 1951–1961 were caused by CVD; the expected number of these total deaths was 60.2, which would include 8.5 for cerebrovascular disease. For pensioners who died 1926–1950, there were 5 CVD deaths vs. 0.8 expected. In addition, for those who died between 1946–1961 while still employed, there were 9 CVD deaths instead of the 5.6 expected, and again this was the only excess noted. I have not found any further evidence to this point, and it would appear to have little impact on the entirety of CVD, but could well be of import in industrial medicine.

A relationship between cadmium in the air and cardiovascular disease death rates was posited by R. E. CARROLL (1966). Fortunate for our purposes, the coefficient of correlation for CVD deaths was not significant (—0.21). We can therefore leave explanations (if any) to the cardiologists.

SCHROEDER (1960) called attention to a positive association between cardiovascular disease death rates and the degree of softness of the municipal water supply. He later (1966) confirmed this finding, with highly significant correlation coefficients for hypertensive heart disease and arteriosclerotic heart disease in both males and females. For cerebrovascular disease the coefficients were —0.25 (P < 0.05) for males and —0.17 (P > 0.05) for females. He noted that there was no significant correlation between the cardiac and CVD geographic distributions.

Confirmation of this thesis was provided by MORRIS (1961) in England for cardiovascular disease as a whole, including CVD, myocardial degeneration, and (in the young) CAD; but *not* for hypertension with or without heart disease. Other ills were not so correlated. He thought (1962) rainfall might also be of import in this relationship.

MULCAHY (1964) was unable to find any significant correlation for any component or age-group of cardiac deaths or CVD deaths in Ireland with water hardness or rainfall.

BIÖRCK (1965) in an investigation of 35 urban areas of Sweden felt he did to some degree confirm the water hypothesis. Significant negative correlations with water hardness though were seldom present for the *major* cardiovascular disease deaths. For CVD, only females age 45—64 (P < 0.01) and males age 65—74 (P < 0.05) showed any noteworthy correlation. Category 422 ("other degenerative heart diseases") more often showed the significant relationships. Among the constituents of the water, only the calcium content seemed to bear a relation with death rates, and now CVD joined the remainder of the common cardiac deaths as showing no significant correlation. However, category 422 did have a generally consistent and significant negative correlation with calcium content, more pronounced than with water hardness. In sum therefore, whatever role water or its constituents may play in certain types of cardiac disease, it seems quite unlikely to be a factor of import in CVD.

References

General

BERKSON   30
BRADSHAW   40
DAVID   71
GIEL   121
JÖRGENSEN   165
MARSHALL   219
MEYER   240, 242
MILLIKAN   245
OSTFELD   275
PAFFENBARGER   279, 280
REUTER   304
STALLONES   336, 337
WELLS   382
WHISNANT   384

Hypertension

ACHESON, R.   2, 3
ADAMS   7
AURELL   21
BALOW   26
BERKSON   30
Commission on Chronic
   Illness   60
DUSTAN*   90
editorial   92
GEIGER   117
GIFFORD, R. W.*   123
HAMILTON*   139
HARINGTON*   144
HOWARD, J.   157
JELLINEK   163
KANNEL   169, 170
KINSEY*   178

KRUEGER   184
KURLAND   188
LEISHMAN*   199
McDOWELL   231
MERRETT   239
MEYER   242
MIALL   243
MOHLER*   252
PAFFENBARGER   277
PAUL, O.   285
ROSE   309, 310
SCHROEDER   318
SCOTCH   321
SMIRK*   330
STAMLER   335
TAKAHASHI   355, 356
THORNER   362
YULE   408
* = treatment studies

CAD and AS

ACHESON, R.   3
BIÖRCK   33
BORHANI   36—38
Commission on Chronic
   Illness   60
DAWBER   73—75
HECHTER   147
HOLMAN   154
KANNEL   171
KATSUKI   172
KURLAND   188
NAIK   265
PAFFENBARGER   278, 281

PELL   287
SKYRING   329
STAMLER   335
UEDA   368
WALKER   378
YANO   402
YOSHITOSHI   406

Cholesterol and fats

CONNOR, W. E.   62
CUMINGS   68
FELDMAN   100
HEYMAN   150
KANNEL   169, 170
KATSUKI   176
McGANDY   232
MEYER   242
NEFZGER   267
ROBINSON   308

Smoking

CROFTON   65
DOLL   83
HAMMOND   140, 141
KAHN   168
KANNEL   170

Other

BICKERSTAFF   32
BIÖRCK   33
CARROLL, R. E.   52
COLE   59
DINGWALL-FORDYCE   80
GIFFORD, A. J.   122

GURDJIAN   135
HARVALD   145
ILLIS   160
JENNETT   163 (1)
KANNEL   170

McDOWELL   231
MEYER   242
MORRIS   260
MULCAHY   262

PELL   288
SCHROEDER   319, 320
SHAFEY   322
STAMLER   335

Chapter X

Changing Times and CVD

This section will be devoted to the question whether the relative components of CVD have been changing over the years, and most particularly to whether there has been a decline in cerebral hemorrhage and an increase in thrombo-embolic CVD.

The question is of course two fold: have the disease-frequencies altered, and have the mortality-rates altered? If the case-fatality rate were the same, a "yes" answer to either would be appropriate to the other, so the question should include the third aspect of a change in case-fatality rates.

The time-interval over which changes can be measured with any degree of accuracy in CVD from mortality data is extremely short. For general purposes information before 1948 is of little value, mostly because of the markedly different coding schemes for the subdivisions of CVD. Mortality statistics early in this century were most often available as a unit which was generally called "cerebral apoplexy" or "cerebral hemorrhage". Subdivisions, when used, incorporated SAH with cerebral hemorrhage, and "cerebral softening" was a category distinct from cerebral thrombosis.

Crude mortality rates for CVD as a whole have of course risen with time as the population has aged. However the age-specific rates do not appear to me to have shown any appreciable change, as the figures in Chapter IV demonstrate. Some workers however consider there has been a real decline in the USA and England for deaths under age 75 attributed to CVD. BERKSON (1965) and BORHANI [1966(2)] associate this with a decline in hypertensive deaths. Even if one classed the modest changes as real, I would be inclined to call upon change in diagnosis rather that change in disease as the most probable explanation. "Sudden death" frequently was attributed to "apoplexy" in early years of this century; now most are called "heart attack".

SAH. While the sum may be constant, the parts could still certainly have changed. For SAH we are limited to the past 20 years or so as the maximum in which deaths would have been coded as such. In an earlier chapter we considered GIEL's study (1965) of SAH in the Netherlands. He claimed to have demonstrated a real increase in deaths from SAH in Rotterdam as well as in the entirety of Holland between 1950 and 1962. The average age-specific mortality rates for the two periods (1950—1954 and 1958—1962) have been drawn in an earlier figure and compared with those for Denmark 1956—1960. Both Netherland series fall well within the Danish confidence limits, and the absolute changes are small. To me this indicates there is no evidence that the mortality rates have truly increased, despite the change in overall crude mortality rates. GIEL also points to an increasing frequency with time of SAH in Rotterdam in either absolute numbers or the proportions of deaths or admissions to hospital. But these changes are by no means consistent. If we compare consecutive years and assign a "+" when the first year is greater than the second, "—" when it is less, and "0" when it is the same, we find the following from his data:

SAH	Year (vs. the next year)									
	1951	1952	1953	1954	1955	1956	1957	1958	1959	1960
Admissions No.	+	—	+	+	—	+	—	—	—	+
Admissions %	+	—	+	+	—	+	0	—	0	+
Hosp. deaths No.	+	—	+	—	—	—	+	+	—	—
Hosp. deaths %	+	—	+	—	—	+	+	+	—	—
City deaths No.	—	+	+	+	—	—	0	—	0	—

A consistent increase would be manifest by all "—" signs. I can discern no real trend in these data. So in general we may conclude there is no good evidence for a change in SAH deaths or cases (and by inference case-fatality rates) in the short time-span under consideration.

Cerebral Hemorrhage. In Chapters VI and VII we pointed out that cerebral hemorrhage comprised some 54 % of CVD deaths during the 1950's among 18 countries according to age-adjusted average annual mortality rates; in turn cerebral thrombosis-embolism was 29%, "other" CVD 14%, and SAH 3%. Since the weighted average annual mortality rate was 99.46, these percentages, in this instance, also represent the respective mortality rates in cases per 100,000 population. We have also shown that the age-specific curves for cerebral hemorrhage, thrombosis, and "other CVD" are in general quite similar in Denmark, and therefore an alteration in age-distribution of the population would be most unlikely to cause any major shift in the overall relative proportions of these respective entities. Cerebral hemorrhage will be considered here in its relationship with cerebral thrombosis, as well as an entity *sui generis*.

From a reassessment of death certificates for 1920—1960 in Memphis, Tennessee, KRUEGER (1967) concluded that, although annual mortality rates for CVD as a whole were essentially constant, cerebral hemorrhage deaths had diminished and cerebral thrombosis had increased dramatically from some 10 to 50 cases per 100,000. The "cerebral hemorrhage" category he used included SAH and some "other" CVD. The concomitant fall in hypertension deaths in the same study has been described by PAFFENBARGER [1966 (1)].

P. C. GORDON (1966) has also pointed out this same coincident trend in decreasing cerebral hemorrhage and hypertension, while cerebral thrombosis deaths increased in Canada between 1950 and 1964. Representative crude mortality rates are as follows:

Year	331	332	334	330—334
1950	55	20	15	91
1955	53	24	11	90
1960	47	27	10	86
1964	41	25	9	78

A similar time differential for hypertensive deaths by race was attributed by
HOWARD (1965) to effective treatment in whites vs. Negroes. For England and
Wales as well as the United States, WYLIE too [1961, 1962 (2)] called attention
to the fall in cerebral hemorrhage deaths and the rise in thrombosis.

The most important study which speaks to changes with time however is that
of YATES (1964, 1966). From official mortality statistics over the prior 30 years
he called attention to a slight decline in cerebral hemorrhage deaths in England
and Wales, while those for thrombosis increased three-fold in this period. For age-
specific rates there was a clear decline in hemorrhage deaths over age 65, and it
was in this same group that thrombosis rose most markedly. His most telling
argument though was where he counted the numbers of autopsied cases of hemorrhage and infarction found in one to three Manchester hospitals from 1926 through
1961, one hospital alone in 1926—1937 and 1941—1946. One of the other two was
apparently a predominantly geriatric hospital. He then compared the autopsied
cases with an expected number of either entity derived from the appropriate
mortality figures from England and Wales, and showed an excellent agreement for
all years between the observed and expected numbers of each. The ratio of thrombosis (i.e. cerebral infarct) to hemorrhage from both sources over the years is
cited below:

Year	CI/CH ratios from		Av. annual change	
	(A) autopsies	(B) mortality statistics	(A) ratio	(B) ratio
1926—1937	0.40*	0.45	—	—
1938—1940	0.47	0.58	0.01	0.02
1941—1946	0.55*	0.63	0.02	0.01
1947—1948	0.64	0.72	0.02	0.02
1949—1950	0.71	0.82	0.04	0.05
1951—1952	0.82	0.97	0.06	0.08
1953—1954	0.97	1.04	0.08	0.03
1955—1956	1.33	1.18	0.18	0.07
1957—1958	1.43	1.30	0.05	0.06
1959—1960	1.18	1.37	— 0.12	0.04
1961	1.48	1.42	0.15	0.05

* single hospital

There are several aspects worthy of note here. 1) Coding of CVD deaths before
about 1948 was tripartite: SAH and cerebral hemorrhage together; "cerebral
thrombosis"; and "cerebral softening"*. 2) Hospital CVD autopsy cases in the

* The ISC nomenclature of the fourth (1929) and fifth (1938) revisions actually had more
than three divisions for CVD, but the three noted above are what were most commonly cited
in the literature. Only the numbered titles, in this instance No. 83 for CVD as a whole, were
obligatory; the lettered subdivisions were optional. In the International List, 83a was "cerebral
(and subarachnoid) haemorrhage", 83b "cerebral embolism and thrombosis", 83c "softening
of the brain", 83d "hemiplegia and other paralyses of unstated origin", and 83e "other intracranial effusions". For use in the United States, 83d and e were combined as No. 83d, defined
as d above. "Cerebral arteriosclerosis" was a disease of the circulatory system (No. 97). CVD
as a whole was also denoted as VI—37 in the Intermediate List and as No. 22 in the Abridged
List of causes of death (Bureau of the Census, 1940).

first period were 12 a year and during the war years were about 35 per annum for 1938–1940 and 15 per annum for 1941–1946. The numbers increased strikingly thereafter to about 200 per annum by 1953 and more slowly to some 270 per annum by 1959. 3) The National Health Service Act was adopted about 1948.

How might these points influence the cited ratios in the mortality statistics? Effects of the new ISC code would cause many more deaths to be coded 332 (cerebral thrombosis-embolism) than under the prior "cerebral thrombosis", as the cases previously ascribed to "cerebral softening" would now be included. Cerebral hemorrhage (331) would now be less as SAH (330) was removed from the category. The *rate* of change in the infarct/hemorrhage ratio through 1948 was slight, at but 0.02 a year. Thereafter the annual rate of change was three times as great. More widespread conformation to proper coding, increased utilization of medical facilities, a rising proportion of hospital deaths (hence autopsies), and better diagnostic standards — all would contribute to an increasing ratio of thrombosis/ hemorrhage deaths in the mortality statistics.

What might similarly influence the hospital ratios, since coding artefact would not be a problem in autopsied cases? First, most of the early data came from one hospital, the Manchester Royal Infirmary. Before and during the war especially hospitalization in this, the major facility, would seem to have been more likely for the acutely ill, and, as will be shown, early deaths are much more common in cerebral hemorrhage than infarction. Even if *cases* were equal in number, a ratio of about 0.5 or so would seem likely from autopsies in a short-term general hospital. The war especially would have restricted admissions to the more grave problems. In the post-war period there would then be expected a return to a wider admission policy, and the socioeconomic changes in Britain (plus the National Health Service) would have promoted hospitalization for many more chronic conditions and many more people. Autopsies would therefore show a decided increase in patients who died *with* cerebral infarction, as well as in those who died *because of* cerebral infarction. Recall that in ARONSON's (1966) New York series $1/4$ of all brains examined in routine autopsy showed encephalomalacia. The addition of a predominantly geriatric facility would greatly accelerate the rates for infarcts in autopsies, and one of YATES' hospitals was such. The dramatic change in this ratio in 1955 is also highly suggestive of some source of input bias; this might have been the opening of an additional geriatric wing, accelerated fatalities among chronic patients who had entered the facilities early in the N.H.S. period, overcrowding with resultant restriction to the more gravely ill, or other possible explanations. After 1955 the thrombosis-hemorrhage ratio fluctuated quite drastically, although the number of cases was the highest then for the entire study. This too suggests some artefact rather than a true reflection of the disease.

YATES' report has been considered in such great detail because it is the single apparently solid basis for the hypothesis that cerebral hemorrhage is truly declining in relation to cerebral thrombosis. Even this extremely careful and well-planned study has, I believe, flaws which are fatal to the acceptance of this hypothesis as having been validated.

AURELL (1964) provides further evidence for the possibility of a true decline in cerebral hemorrhage deaths in Sweden; the rates do not differ significantly however between the early and later periods (Table VII—a—4). He thought that the decline in his study was in those *under* 65, unlike the English results.

Thus we may conclude from mortality data that while there might possibly be a true albeit modest decrease in deaths attributed to cerebral hemorrhage, the admixture of custom and coding errors makes this difficult to prove. We may recall that "apoplexy" and cerebral hemorrhage" were in the early part of this century the officially sanctioned epithets for CVD as a whole. The time-lag of adherence to new regulations undoubtedly has caused an unknown number of thrombotic deaths (332) to be coded as hemorrhage (331). In addition there is some misinformation, even among the experts, that unqualified terms such as "apoplexy", "cerebro-vascular accident", or "stroke" *should* be coded as 331, instead of as the correct 334, "other CVD" (see Chapter II).

Cerebral Thrombosis. The changes in cerebral thrombosis are even more difficult to evaluate. The studies of interest have already been cited. Thrombosis deaths have increased not only with declining hemorrhage, but also with declining "other CVD". A goodly portion of the change in this "new" category of thrombosis is likely to be diagnostic fashion. And yet, the increase *seems* too marked to attribute with assurance to this point. In addition, the increase is also apparent within any given age-group in England (YATES). It therefore seems *likely* that there has been a true increase in cerebral thrombosis-embolism death reports in recent years. Even if we accept this point though, the question arises whether this is attributable to better diagnosis. Cerebral hemorrhage is usually catastrophic with early death; in cerebral thrombosis, early fatality rates are notably less, and the time of death — as will be seen — is prolonged after the ictus. It is certainly reasonable to assume that at least *some* of the "true" increase in CVD deaths due to thrombosis is a resultant of greater diagnostic acumen or more careful coding. Thus we leave *sub judice* whether cerebral thrombosis is indeed an illness of increasing frequency.

If the data from mortality statistics are of use for only a short time span, those from population surveys might be considered instantaneous. We therefore have no useful information on the frequency of CVD as an illness over time, nor of course of its components. While numbers can be sought from hospitals series to this point, they must be considered far too biased to be of use. For example, in one major city teaching hospital in New York, Bellevue, GROCH (1961) recorded but 7% of CVD were cerebral hemorrhage in the 1956—1960 period. At another major city teaching hospital in New York, Kings County, the vast majority of patients admitted with stroke were cerebral hemorrhage in 1952 (personal observation). We therefore have no basis for assessing whether the frequency of occurrence of cerebral hemorrhage or thrombosis is changing with time, and therefore no evidence for changes in the case-fatality rates. As indicated, even the mortality statistics do not indicate unequivocally any real change in frequency of CVD deaths, in whole or in part. We can also recall from Chapter VI, our estimate of "true" proportions of CVD types to be expected, based on population survey frequencies and early case-fatality rates. The expected frequencies for mortality data were SAH, 8%; cerebral hemorrhage, 30%; cerebral thrombosis 50% (a ratio of 1.67); and "other CVD" 12%. These proportions are quite similar to the most recent England-Wales data, and would possibly support the thesis that changes in thrombosis-hemorrhage are indeed merely coding artefacts.

References

ARONSON 18
AURELL 21
BERKSON 30
BORHANI 36

Bureau of the Census 48
GIEL 121
GORDON, P. C. 128
GROCH 131, 132

HOWARD, J. 157
PAFFENBARGER 277
WYLIE 396, 397
YATES 403, 404

Chapter XI

The Course of CVD

It is of obvious import to know what the future will bring the patient with a stroke, or at least how groups of patients are likely to fare. In this context we are of course limited to those sources which provide a potential for follow-up information: hospital series and population surveys. It may be obvious by now that I look on many hospital data with a jaundiced eye, but for this aspect we are unfortunately very limited in the amount of information available from the population studies. It is apparent that we cannot describe a "natural history of stroke" — even by considering the components separately. Since all our information is happily provided by physicians, we must speak of the "natural history of the variably treated patients with stroke", and make some attempt at least to think of the separate portions of this phrase.

All CVD. Since it is likely that "other" CVD is in fact largely cerebral thrombosis-embolism, since from our previous data cerebral hemorrhage cannot be separated from thrombosis by age or sex in the living or the dead, and since SAH is such a small fraction of CVD, it is perhaps valid to begin this discussion by consideration of the course of CVD as a whole. While disability is a major feature with these ills, we will restrict our attention to the apparently simple question of survival over time. Further, we shall cite our deaths as cumulative case-fatality rates with time, that is, the cumulative percentage of the original group who have died by the end of the designated period. No attempt will be made to assign a cause of death or to take note of related ills. Similarly there will be no life-table analysis; the only concession to mathematical manipulation will be the presentation of the cumulative fatality rates against a logarithmic scale for time, and this only because the figures then are easier to graph.

Our three general sources of information on the course of the disease are 1) survivors of the ictus who are hospitalized, primarily for special study or rehabilitation, 2) hospital series per se, chiefly from the acute-care institutions, and 3) population surveys, really limited to EISENBERG's (1964) study of Middlesex, Connecticut.

In Table XI–1 are listed cumulative fatality rates from these sources for all CVD combined. For the first part, ADAMS (1967) and KATZ (1966) studied patients in this country who had survived the stroke but were in need of rehabilitation. MARSHALL's patients in London (1959) were primarily referred because of his special interest in stroke. FELGER (1961) in Vienna would appear to have also been at a referral point, since a goodly proportion of patients were a year or more after their stroke when seen. These series seem to split in this fashion for course also; for the rehabilitation patients, fatality rates were some 20% by six months and 60% by four years. The referral centers reached 20% after two years and 40% in four. For comparison, the early survivors of the ictus in the population study of EISENBERG had a cumulative fatality rate of 66% in five years. The difference between the rehabilitation and the referral sources might well represent those between patients with major residua and without. The population survey rate resembles that of the former group.

We should obtain a better idea of the true course from the B. series. Here we can see that about one in three stroke patients is dead in two months and about half within two years. Conversely EISENBERG's study would indicate half the patients die within two *weeks* and three-fourths in one year. By five years 85%

Table XI–1. *Cumulative case-fatality rates, all CVD*
Cumulative rate in percentages to end of:

Source	N	Av. Age	1 wk	2 wk	1 mo	2 mo	6 mo	1 yr	2 yr	3 yr	4 yr	5 yr
A. Survivors of the ictus												
ADAMS (1967) total	710	69				19					53	
male	314	70				19					50	
female	396	69				19					56	
FELGER (1961)	1000	63						8	19	31	40	45
KATZ (1966)	159	71					20	31	48	55	60	64
MARSHALL (1959)	248	59						7	17	28	40	48
EISENBERG (1964)	83	73										66
B. Hospital Series												
BOYLE (1965)	477	68	c. 10		31	47						
CARROLL (1962)	98	67	20		37		48	51	60			
CONANT (1965) total	254	c. 70				32		40	45	53		
male	111	c. 67				26		33	40	49		
female	143	c. 72				36		45	49	56		
HOWARD (1963)	97	68					35	41	53			
MOUREN (1965) total	489	c. 65	13	19	24	26						
male	255	—	9	15	20	24						
female	234	—	17	23	28	30						
C. Population Survey												
EISENBERG (1964)	191	74	42	50	57		67	72		81		85

had expired. One explanation for this discrepancy is the age of the patients at ictus. In this last group the average age was 74, while the hospital series were some five years younger. While this might not seem much of a difference, when we divide the Middlesex cases according to age, we see there is indeed a striking variation with age in the case-fatality rates (Fig. XI–1). The data are in Appendix Table XI–a–1. Similar differences were apparent in FELGER's study (1961). In CARROLL's work (1962), the fatality rate for those under age 51 was 38%. This rose steadily in the succeeding decades as 54, 59, and 61%, and for those over age 80, the case-fatality rate was 83%, all in accord with the Middlesex experience. The Middlesex data further suggest that the rate of death after the ictus does not depend upon age but that the proportion who die is strongly age-dependent

(Table XI–a–1). In other words age has no bearing on the *length* of survival after stroke, but it has a very marked effect on the *fact* of survival.

SAH. The principal source also for the course of SAH must be the massive Cooperative Aneurysm Study to which other data may be related [LOCKSLEY,

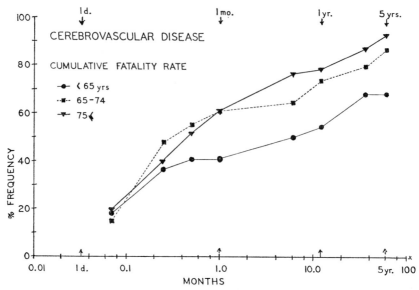

Fig. XI–1. Cumulative case-fatality rates as percentages against time (on a logarithmic scale) for all CVD from Connecticut population survey according to age at ictus. Data are in Appendix Table XI–a–1, from EISENBERG (1964)

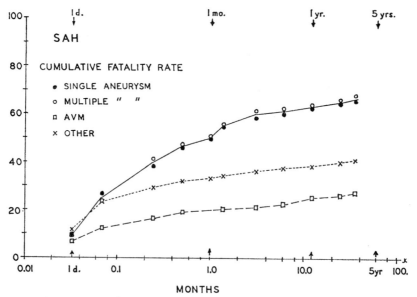

Fig. XI–2. Cumulative case-fatality rates as in XI–1 for SAH according to cause. Data are in Appendix Table XI–a–2, from LOCKSLEY (1966)

1966 (1, 2, 4)]. In Fig. XI—2 are plotted cumulative fatality rates, for which the information may be found in Appendix Table XI—a—2. The rates are for the first bleed for aneurysm, AVM, and "other" SAH, in patients who were *not* subjected to surgery. They may therefore be weighted against the "good-risk" patients for later course, and overrepresented by "poor risk" patients in the early deaths.

Table XI—2. *Major causes and course of subarachnoid hemorrhage (SAH) from the Cooperative Study* (LOCKSLEY)

Cause	Frequency Percent	Mean Age	Case-Fatality Rate* (percent)	I-C hem (%)**
Aneurysm only	51	52	59	90***
Arteriovenous malformation only	6	38	22	?
Hypertension and/or Arteriosclerosis	15	59	75	88
Hypertension (HT)	5	55	51	89
HT and AS	8	60	92	90
Arteriosclerosis (AS)	2	64	73	78
"Idiopathic"	22	49	18	77
Miscellaneous	6	—	—	—
Total	100	52	44	—

   * in first three months, cumulative rate
  ** percent of fatal cases with intracerebral hemorrhage
*** percent of acute deaths

Table XI—3. *Frequency of intracerebral hemorrhage in patients with SAH who died or survived (3 months), according to diagnosis, from the Cooperative Study* (LOCKSLEY)

		% with I-C hem.	N	Mean age
Aneurysm (deaths in 72 hours)		90	104	(52)
Aneurysm-survivors		?	—	(52)
AVM total		?	—	38
SAH with HT	— deaths	89	78	57
	— survivors	11	75	54
SAH with HT and AS	— deaths	90	204	59
	— survivors	24	17	62
SAH with AS	— deaths	78	41	67
	— survivors	0	15	55
Idiopathic SAH	— deaths	77	62	55
	— survivors	6	286	48

The rates for single vs. multiple aneurysms however are essentially identical, and surgical intervention would be less likely for the bulk of these. Therefore this should be a reasonable approximation to the spontaneous course of SAH patients who reach hospital.

    Further information on the early course of SAH is set forth in Table XI—2. The case-fatality rate within three months is noted for the major causes: for aneurysm it is 59% and for AVM 22%. "Idiopathic" SAH has a cumulative fatality rate of 18%. Most ominous are SAH with cardiovascular disease. With hypertension 51%; with arteriosclerosis 73%; and with both together, 92% are dead by three months after the hemorrhage. Of great interest here is the last column. For those who died, regardless of age or cause, 80 to 90% had intracerebral hemorrhage in association with the subarachnoid bleed.

In contrast, those who survived had evidence of intracerebral hemorrhage in 0 to 24% (Table XI–3). The frequency for intracerebral hemorrhage among the aneurysm deaths is among those who died within the first 72 hours, and I could find no comparable information for AVM cases [PERRET, 1966 (2)].

Table XI–4. *Percentage frequency distribution of early deaths (within 72 hours) from SAH with aneurysm by site of aneurysm (single bleeding aneurysms only*) from the Cooperative Study* (LOCKSLEY) *compared with London experience* (McKISSOCK)

Site	Deaths	All such aneurysms	London-Σ
Internal Carotid	22.1	37.7	35.5
Middle Cerebral	30.8	20.8	23.2
Ant. Communicating	33.7	30.3	32.8
distal Ant. Cerebral	4.8	2.8	3.3
Basilar	2.9 ⎫	2.9 ⎫	⎫
Cerebellar	1.9 ⎬ 8.6	0.8 ⎬ 8.5	⎬ 5.2
Other	3.8 ⎭	4.8 ⎭	⎭
Total	100.0	100.1	100.0
N	104	2349	1455
% with 1-C hem.**	90%	?	?

* 20% of aneurysms were multiple
** intracerebral (and 9 intracerebellar) hemorrhage, plus one subdural

Acute deaths with aneurysm are more common in middle cerebral aneurysms and less common in those of the internal carotid region than expected, probably because of the greater tendency of the former to bleed into the parenchyma (Table XI–4).

The involved subject of treatment vs. course of aneurysms is discussed by the authors listed *in extenso* in the references. Most of these are surgical series with little attempt to obtain comparable data for non-operated but operable cases. Especially noteworthy however are the papers of McKISSOCK (1960, 1962, 1964, 1965) who did try to evaluate therapy in a rather well-controlled fashion. In posterior communicating and middle-cerebral lesions — but not anterior communicating — his surgical series did notably better than the conservatively treated. POOL (1966) disputes his pessimistic view on the surgical results in anterior communicating aneurysms. The conservatively-treated aneurysm patients from the Cooperative Study are discussed by NISHIOKA (1966). SAHS [1966 (2)] gave a negative evaluation of hypothermia in the management of the acutely ill, though he thought hypotensive therapy might be of use. The AVM cases of the Cooperative Study were described by PERRET [1966 (2)]. The evaluation of their course is complicated by surgical intervention, early vs. late deaths, bleeding vs. non-bleeding AVM, AVM with and without fits, and AVM with and without intracerebral hematomas. Operations varied from cervical ligation to resection. PERRET too apparently seemed to leave open the question of who should be treated in what fashion.

Cerebral Hemorrhage. Good information on the course of intracerebral hemorrhage in recent years is sparse. PENNYBACKER (1963) mentioned his modest success in the surgical evacuation of intracerebral hematoma in such cases. Better results though were reported by ARSENI (1967) with this operation. Personal experience in a large city hospital some years ago led me to believe that only the unusual patient with massive intracerebral hemorrhage would survive. Obviously not every hemorrhage is massive however. TENNENT (1949) in Wisconsin reported a very low case-fatality rate of 29% in 75 patients, and these comprised $3/_4$ of his CVD cases. Only two of his 27 with cerebral thrombosis succumbed. This seems a surprisingly benign experience for a state general hospital. KELLY in England is cited by WHISNANT (1966) as giving a case-fatality rate of 91% from a general hospital, which is more what I would have expected. Without fear of contradiction therefore, we can fall back upon the experience of EISENBERG (1964) in Middlesex, Connecticut, as noted here for his 68 cerebral hemorrhage patients averaging 73 years of age at ictus:

	Cumulative fatality rate to end of:						
Time	1 wk	2 wk	1 mo	6 mo	1 yr	3 yr	5 yr
Rate (%)	59	75	82	87	87	91	97

An unspecified but presumably small number of SAH were included here. Note the very early accumulation of deaths. Within two weeks 3 out 4 patients were dead and nearly 9 out of 10 within a few months. Thus KELLY's data would appear reasonable. The cumulative rates from Middlesex are drawn in Fig. XI–3, where they are compared with the course for cerebral thrombosis cases in the same study. Unlike the course by age at ictus for all strokes, these patients show a highly significant difference in the *intervals* at which deaths accumulate in hemorrhage vs. thrombosis (Appendix Table XI–a–3), while the ultimate five-year fatality rate is quite similar. Of course a comparison of *early* deaths would show a significant difference in rate between hemorrhage and thrombosis. Here then we do have some documentation for the thesis presented early that mortality rate comparisons between hemorrhage and thrombosis would be biased by both the relative case-fatality rates *per se* and the smaller chances of retrieval of late deaths (and hence of thrombosis cases).

Cerebral Thrombosis. Papers on the course of thromboembolic stroke are many, and only what seem to me to be the major ones in each of our source-categories will be displayed in any detail, while a positive attempt will be made also to avoid those which are evaluations of specific treatment, whether surgical or medical. Table XI–5 summarizes the data.

JOHN MARSHALL's early study (1959) has been alluded to under the first section of this chapter. Of these 248 British patients referred to him, 167 were classed as cerebral thrombosis. He later (1961) reported a similar prospective study, with case-fatality rates identical to the prior one. For comparative purpose we may include in this category A (survivors of the ictus) the appropriate proportions of cases from the studies of ROBINSON (1959) and PINCOCK (1957). It may be seen that in three of these works only 5% of survivors died in the first year, but this rate increased steadily to almost half the cases within five years after ictus. In ROBINSON's series the cumulative fatality rates were regularly about twice as high as the others for the first three years, but age at ictus was 10 years greater (68)

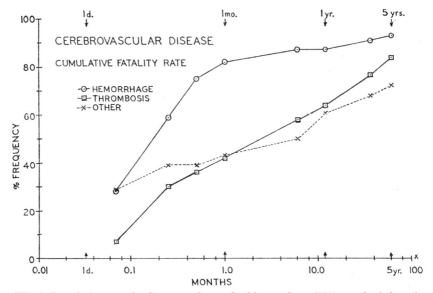

Fig. XI–3. Cumulative case-fatality rates for cerebral hemorrhage (331), cerebral thrombosis-embolism (332), and other CVD (334), from Connecticut population survey. Data are in Appendix Table XI–a–3, from EISENBERG (1964)

than in MARSHALL's group. PINCOCK's survivors may have been of a similarly young age. This was not spelled out in his paper and I cited the age for the total group.

The hospital series include the studies of LINDGREN (1958) in Göteborg, Sweden, GURDJIAN (1961) in Detroit, McDOWELL (1961) in New York, and ROBINSON (1959) in Worcester, Massachusetts. Two reports from veterans hospitals in Winnipeg, Canada (PINCOCK, 1957) and in North Carolina (DAVID, 1960) are also included; in this last about $1/_3$ of cases were from the associated University Hospital. While early rates are rather variable, by six months one in four patients had died; and by two years better than one in three had succumbed. Between $1/_2$ and $2/_3$ were dead by the end of five years. The heaviest fatality rates were seen in the study of ROBINSON (1959), and his patients were also clearly the eldest with an average age of 69 at ictus. Further evidence that age is a major factor in the course is indicated by the case-fatality rate of but one (WELLS, 1961) or two (LOUIS, 1966) per cent in patients under age 50.

Returning once again to EISENBERG's study (1964) we see the notably higher fatality rates in each period. One in three died early, half were dead by six months and two-thirds by one year. The cumulative fatality rate after five years was 84%. This is not necessarily as discrepant from the hospital results as it appears, since his patients were on the average 75 years old when they suffered their stroke.

We may compare in McDOWELL's series (1961) the course for carotid system and basilar-vertebral thromboses. The rates look quite similar, and this is confirmed in formal analysis (Appendix Table XI—a—4), despite the author's contention they do differ.

Table XI–5. *Cumulative fatality rates, cerebral thrombosis*

Source	Special features	N	Av. age	Cumulative rate in percent to end of:									
				1 wk	2 wk	1 mo	2 mo	6 mo	1 yr	2 yr	3 yr	4 yr	5 yr
A. Survivors of the ictus													
ROBINSON		737	68.1						17	28	42	48	58
MARSHALL (prospective)		177	58.2						6	16			
PINCOCK	VAH	101	(64)						4	18	25	36	45
MARSHALL	(referral)	167	(59)						5	13	23	34	44
B. Hospital series													
LINDGREN		65	42.7			11		22		34			38
GURDJIAN		98	56.3			4	6						42
DAVID	VAH	87	57.3				11		29	38			
McDOWELL		107	60.2			21		27	29	35			
Mc DOWELL	carotid	57	59.0			25		26	26	32			
Mc DOWELL	basilar	50	61.6			16		28	32	38			
PINCOCK	VAH	117	63.5					14	18	29	35	44	52
ROBINSON		933	69.0					21	34	43	54	59	67
C. Population surveys													
EISENBERG		91	75.4	30	36	42		58	64		77		84

Treatment of thrombotic stroke, as stated, is not in our province. The major works in which anticoagulant therapy is considered are those of BAKER (1962), ENGER (1965), C. M. FISHER [1961 (1)], GROCH [1961 (1, 2)], HOWELL (1964), McDEVITT (1958), McDOWELL (1965), MILLIKAN (1961), and UDALL (1967). The consensus seems to be that these agents have no value in completed stroke, though some (e.g. FISHER, UDALL), believe they are of value in stroke-in-evolution. While on the topic, BAKER, FISHER, GROCH, HOWELL, and MILLIKAN deal also with anticoagulants in transient ischemic attacks, as do BAKER (1966), PEARCE (1965), and MARSHALL (1965). There does seem to be some evidence these drugs will reduce the frequency of TIA episodes, but I do not believe the authors have yet demonstrated that in TIA patients the frequency of later fatal or non-fatal strokes is altered by their administration. In the treatment of cerebral embolism, the value of anticoagulants seems well established (HOWELL, 1964; McDEVITT, 1958; WELLS, 1959).

Operative intervention is considered by DORNDORF (1965), R. G. FISHER (1961), GURDJIAN (1961, 1965, 1967), HARDIN (1966), HEYMAN (1967), LYONS (1965),

MURPHEY (1965), OJEMANN (1966), THOMPSON (1966, 1967), and YOUNG (1964); ROB (1967) discussed its role in TIA. While it certainly is more esthetically pleasing to have clean pipes rather than clogged ones, I believe the early enthusiasm for surgery on the carotid artery has waned. Certainly it has no role in the *treatment* of completed stroke, and its value in prevention of further episodes is, I think, not solidly established. Too often too there are multiple vessels involved angiographically. Indeed not even cerebral perfusion is improved by this procedure in carotid artery disease, according to O'BRIEN (1967). My *guess* is that the procedure should be considered in otherwise healthy young patients with symptomatic stenosis but not occlusion of the internal carotid in the neck.

MARSHALL [1964 (2)] published data which suggest that reduction of blood pressure in hypertensive stroke patients may prevent further episodes. MEYER (1965) stopped his study of streptokinase when it was found the patients were doing worse than the controls. MARMORSTON (1965) presented preliminary evidence which suggested that Premarin^R *might* have some effect in reducing the frequency of later strokes; the defect is not with the study but with the numbers, which are far too small for confidence. Unfortunately, the results of the Veterans Administration Cooperative Study (1966) would indicate no value for this agent in preventing cerebral infarct, TIA, or myocardial infarct at essentially the same dosage as MARMORSTON used, which was sufficient to cause feminizing side effects in 40% of the patients — and "similar side effects" in 14% of the placebo-treated patients. The latest effort, as yet unproven, is double therapy with diguanides added (FEARNLEY, 1967).

HEYMAN (1966) was able to demonstrate neurologic improvement in some patients with stroke by the use of hyperbaric oxygenation. But only 2 of 22 showed sustained "dramatic" recovery; one was a presumed embolus of 5 hours' duration, and the other an angiographic complication of 2½ hours' duration. Transient improvement was noted in 8; this was "dramatic" in two with emboli of one and two hours' duration, and in the other six was less marked (duration of episodes 1½ to 4 hours in five, 8 days in one). There was no demonstrable neurologic change in the other 12 whose episodes ranged from 2 hours to 1 month in duration.

References

"Stroke"
ADAMS 7, 8
BOYLE 39
CARROLL, D. 51
CONANT 61
EISENBERG 93
FORD 114
HOWARD, F. A. 156
KATZ 177
MARSHALL 222
MERRETT 239
MOUREN 261

SAH
AF BJÖRKESTEN 12
AHMED* 13

ASK-UPMARK 20
COOK* 63
DU BOULAY 87
DUNSMORE 89
GERMAN* 119
GIBBS* 120
GIEL 121
LOCKSLEY 203—206
MAGEE 210
McKISSOCK* 234—237
McMURTRY 238
NISHIOKA 270
PERRET 291, 292
POOL* 297
RICHARDSON* 305
SAHS 313—315

SARNER 316, 317
SVEIN 352, 353
TINDALL* 363
TRUMPY 366
UIHLEIN 369
WALTON 380
WOLF, G. 390
WOLF, G. A. 391
* = surgical treatment series

Cb. H.
ARSENI 19
EISENBERG 93
PENNYBACKER 290
TENNENT 359
WHISNANT 384

Cb. thr.
BAKER 23—25
DAVID 71
DORNDORF 84
EISENBERG 93
ENGER 95
FEARNLEY 98
FISHER, C. M. 104
FISHER, R. G. 110
GROCH 131, 132
GURDJIAN 133—136
HARDIN 143

HEYMAN 149, 151
HOWELL 158
LINDGREN 201
LYONS 209
MARMORSTON 215
MARSHALL 217—222
McDEVITT 228
McDOWELL 230, 231
MEYER 241
MILLIKAN 244
MURPHEY 264

O'BRIEN 271
OJEMANN 272
PINCOCK 294
ROB 306
ROBINSON 307
THOMPSON 360, 361
UDALL 367
Veterans Administration
  Study 374
WELLS 382
YOUNG 407

CHAPTER XII

CVD-Comments and Conclusions

To bring together this mass of data is a difficult chore, but one which I believe is due the reader. Here more than anywhere else in this work should the buyer beware. These are personal interpretations only, and they often differ from published orthodoxy, whether lay or medical. We might begin though with a less controversial aspect, and that is to look at the ISC coding of diseases and deaths referable to CVD (World Health Organization, 1957).

A Suggested Code for CVD. Some gratuitous advice for CVD reclassification might be in order. The relative unreliability of current mortality data would indeed be an asset here, since entrenched positions could more easily be dislodged. I cannot stress too much how important is the potential for information on human disease from morbidity and mortality data, properly classified and encoded. This is an almost untapped resource. And its value will ultimately stand or fall with the individual physician. I would think that a well-designed code could— and should — provide the basis for the presentation of disease in medical school; that this should be so firmly ingrained in the physician's *corpus scientiae* that he will use an ISC number as readily as a hyphenated teutonic eponym. If the doctor works in this fashion, the lay encoders will have a much easier job — and a happier result. The ultimate beneficiary is the individual patient and physician, for the more we know about disease the more effective should be our management. In this day of ultra-structure and twisted helices (or helixes, if you prefer), here is a major contribution each of us can make.

In respect to a new CVD code, I would first of all remove subarachnoid hemorrhage from the category, for reasons to be noted. I would further delete hypertensive encephalopathy from the current "other and ill-defined" CVD class and reassign it exclusively to one of the hypertensive disease categories; my own inclination would be that of essential malignant hypertension (code 445), and no other. The category of cerebral artery spasm should be discarded.

Most importantly though, I would unequivocally and irrevocably make cerebral hemorrhage mean cerebral hemorrhage, and under no circumstances include therein equivalent terms that might be mistaken for this but are indeed non-specific as to the type of CVD intended. Subdural hematoma too should be removed, regardless of no history of trauma.

With these points then, a proposed scheme for coding of CVD deaths and diseases might look like this:

	Type	New ISC No.
(1)	cerebral hemorrhage	331
(2)	cerebral arterial thrombosis (and all equivalents)	332
(3)	cerebral embolism	333

	Type	New ISC No.
(4)	transient ischemic attacks	334
(5)	spinal thrombosis or hemorrhage	335
(6)	cerebral arteriosclerosis, general	336
(7)	cerebral venous thrombosis, non-pyogenic (includes venous sinuses)	337
(8)	CVD, not elsewhere classified	338

Total CVD = 331—338. All categories to be mutually exclusive.

As to SAH, we might codify this as follows:

	Type	New ISC No.
(1)	SAH associated with aneurysm	358
(2)	SAH, other non-traumatic	359

The problem of residua of stroke is less easy to solve. The current rule is that they are classed as CVD in death statistics, but as "other cerebral paralysis" (352) in morbidity statistics. I would think simplicity would require their remaining under CVD for all purposes; perhaps a subcoding as "residua of" (e.g.: 331.1, residua of cerebral hemorrhage) would be a convenient method.

The questions of "underlying cause of death", "associated diseases", and multiple disease coding and retrieval are all under active consideration by the experts, to whom we shall all defer.

Geographic Distribution of CVD. The geography of CVD within countries we could investigate directly *only* from mortality data and *only* for CVD as a whole. In this fashion the entities behaved as if there were no important environmental factor(s) influencing their distribution. International comparisons of all CVD deaths also indicate a quite striking uniformity, especially once we discard from contention the data for Japan and for US Negroes. We must consider though how valid are these statements for the components of CVD, where we have no basis for comparison in similar fashion.

First, SAH: from international mortality statistics (even of Japan), deaths are rather uniformly distributed throughout the world wherever there is useful information. Cases and causes would appear generally to be of the same magnitude in the United States, Great Britain, and Scandinavia. The studies of all CVD deaths *within* countries cannot speak to this point, since SAH is such a small fraction thereof. The limited information otherwise available though does indicate no evidence for geographic (or racial) variation in SAH.

Cerebral hemorrhage + thrombosis + unknown CVD must I believe be considered a single entity in mortality data. Proportions vary so widely in short intervals among otherwise comparable countries, that I cannot but believe the numbers presented in any subgroup are totally unreliable. This was one reason I made no attempt to look at local geographic distributions by type; the other was that the data were unavailable. Scandinavian statistics are generally excellent; indeed I think these countries provide a remarkable epidemiologic resource. Careful recording, small and homogeneous populations, and state-oriented medical care make their information of great value. Further, this appears to be a position of many years' standing in these lands. With all this, cerebral hemorrhage deaths currently cited for Scandinavia are, I believe, grossly inflated. Remember that "stroke" meant "cerebral hemorrhage"early in this century. Then we had "hemorrhage", "thrombosis", and "softening"; and only recently our 4-division code, which is however widely misinterpreted so that "hemorrhage" is *still* a repository for unclassified CVD in many hands.

My guess is that—exclusive of SAH—cerebral hemorrhage is about $1/3$ of all CVD deaths and about $1/5$ of all CVD cases; and that nearly $9/10$ of the remainder are cerebral thrombosis. From mortality data then we have in essence "all CVD" = "hemorrhage" plus "thrombosis", but in a marriage that cannot be dissolved. *If* the true proportions are actually near one hemorrhage to two thromboses, then I think it is highly likely that conclusions for the whole are valid for the parts — unless one posits a reciprocal relationship between them, for which I know no evidence. The reason is that either one by itself is a large enough part of the whole to influence the results in an obvious fashion if its behaviour were grossly different. I believe then that statements pertaining to the geographic distribution of "all CVD" are equally pertinent to cerebral hemorrhage and to cerebral thrombosis.

If this be true, then cerebral hemorrhage *and* thrombosis are *also* not related to geographically-determined environmental factors, but rather occur quite uniformly within and among countries where we have good data.

While these conclusions are indirect, and are based on mortality statistics about which there must always be some question, the available information from hospital series in the United States, Great Britain, Germany, Austria, France, and Scandinavia is really quite comparable in distribution, frequency, sex, and age among these lands. Population studies of several parts of the United States and Britain, and Australia, also provide no evidence of differences in relative or absolute frequency. Similar age-distributions for each in all lands would also imply no notable variations. The major demonstrable difference between cerebral hemorrhage and thrombosis would seem to be in their early case-fatality rates. Therefore I believe that cerebral hemorrhage and cerebral thrombosis too are diseases without apparent exogenous features.

Sex Ratios. CVD as a whole shows essentially equal occurrence in males and females regardless of age or location. Cerebral hemorrhage too appears of equal frequency. There is *possibly* a slight excess of males in young patients with thrombosis, but equal rates in the elderly. One component of cerebral thrombosis and one of SAH do show sex-related differences, reasons for which totally escape me. In the former, TIA is reported twice as often in males. In the latter, females predominate to a lesser extent (about 1.4 to 1) in aneurysmal SAH, but are even more in excess for aneurysms of the internal carotid region; further they were generally 9 years older than the males at the time of the bleed. Other types of SAH were quite uniform by sex in age and frequency. With these exceptions then, CVD appears a state of equal risk by sex as well as by geography.

SAH is not CVD. Resons for including SAH in "stroke" are not clear to me, other than early coding custom when this category was incorporated in cerebral hemorrhage. Then too, it is a group of disorders recently separated from the remainder of intracranial hemorrhage. Certainly in clinical behavior, in causes, in age-distribution — this group is in no way similar to the remainder of CVD. Since angiomas are coded elsewhere, a basis in their being ultimately vascular seems insufficient. As mentioned early in this Chapter, I would much favor removing this from the categories for CVD.

Race and CVD. To me, one of the most intriguing findings in this whole work is the inadequacy of the evidence for the dogma of racial susceptibility in CVD. Indeed, as covered extensively in Chapter VIII, the weight of evidence is that there is *no* racial predilection for CVD in US Negroes or in Japan. The startling findings from the population survey in Hisayama and the autopsy results in Hiroshima and Nagasaki do I believe negate completely the purported high frequency of CVD and especially cerebral hemorrhage deaths in Japan.

I would perhaps go further, and venture the prediction that a reported high frequency of CVD deaths (especially when the excess is in "hemorrhage" and "other" CVD) will be found to correlate with a scarcity of medical facilities (physicians and hospitals), in either numbers or utilization. Local distributions in the United States, Denmark, Norway, and Sweden — and even in Japan — suggest this is so. Rates in a given land (U.S., South Africa) appear higher for those racial or ethnic groups that one might expect would have less adequate medical care. In Japan of course this is far from the entire answer, and diagnostic customs and tradition there, I surmise, are largely responsible for the massive excess of deaths attributed to CVD, while low autopsy rates would have prevented their discovery.

Related Factors. Aside from race and sex, which do not appear in fact to be major variables in most portions of CVD, there are a number of purported precipitants or concomitants of stroke. It seems to me that hypertension, coronary artery disease, and thromboembolic CVD are (at least) three essentially unrelated entities. Hypertension is a prerequisite (almost) for cerebral hemorrhage. In nonhemorrhagic stroke, there would appear to be some association with hypertension, and perhaps smoking and diabetes. These are low order relationships to which only a small proportion of stroke could be attributed. I say "low-order" for hypertension because its high prevalence in the stroke-ages makes the association (grounded in prospective studies) rather less meaningful. As to CAD, again its high frequency and its common origin in atherosclerosis in general make quite uncertain any specific relationship with CVD. Other factors, such as constituents of blood lipids or drinking water, are inadequately documented as associated features in stroke. Of interest is the limited evidence that genetic factors may well be of import in CVD.

Stroke, Age, and Implications. The most dramatic aspect of CVD — and henceforth we are ignoring SAH — is its relationship with age. As we have seen, both hemorrhage and thrombosis become strikingly more common the older the group in question. Major differences in prognosis for thrombosis are also strongly age-related. ZUMOFF (1966) considered that case-fatality rates were logarithmically related with age in such discrepant states as myocardial infarction, cirrhosis, and cancer. He thought these differing rates each represented an acceleration of the intrinsic human aging process. KOHN (1963) pointed out that "Human aging is characterized by a logarithmic increase in death rate", citing, *inter alia*, atherosclerosis and hypertension as states which show this kind of logarithmic change in frequency with age.

In Fig. XII–1 we have age distributions of three entities from the same autopsy series (ARONSON, 1964). These are the frequency of cerebral vascular occlusions by age, the frequency of areas of encephalomalacia, and the frequency of autopsies. The occlusions and softenings move together, as one would expect. There were 256 persons with occlusions in 4000 autopsies, and in one out of four autopsies encephalomalacia was found. Therefore one curve is not merely a reiteration of another. Of particular interest is the relation of the CVD-curve (occlusions and softenings) to the autopsy-curve. While frequencies differ somewhat by age, the general configuration is quite similar, raising the question whether the "aging process", whatever that might be, is common to all.

We have one last figure (XII—2) to observe. Here we see plotted the total age-specific mortality rates by sex for 1851 and for 1951 in England and Wales,

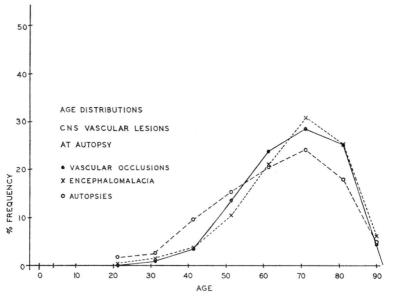

Fig. XII—1. Percentage frequency distributions by age for cerebral vascular occlusions, encephalomalacia, and autopsies from a general hospital. Data are in Appendix Table XII—a—1, from ARONSON (1966)

superimposed (at a 10 to 1 scale) on our oft-presented line representing CVD deaths in the United States and England-Wales. Data are shown in Appendix Table XII—a—2, from TAYLOR (1964). There are several features of interest here. First, the early general mortality rates were equal in both sexes, whereas at present male rates are notably in excess of female. Second, the dramatic change in mortality rates over the past century has been in those under 55 years of age, but male rates above 55 are the same now as before. Third, the slope of the total death rates in the 1800's for the elderly is nearly the slope of current CVD death rates. And this slope is now approximated by the death rates of *all* individuals of both sexes over age 25 or 35.

This raises one (unproven) bifid hypothesis: 1) As we remove treatable deaths we approach the rate of dying intrinsic to the human aging process. 2) The intrinsic aging process results in an age-specific mortality rate whose slope is the same as the age — specific CVD mortality rate. In other words, if this view is correct, stroke — meaning cerebral hemorrhage and thrombosis — may have to be looked upon as a concomitant of aging. As such, it would appear to be preventable only to the extent that we could reverse the aging process. The evidence suggests to me that hemorrhage and thrombosis are indeed "endogenous" rather than "exogenous" diseases. There is nothing apparent in the macroclimate that can be manipulated to alter their frequency. Even in the microclimate, while treating

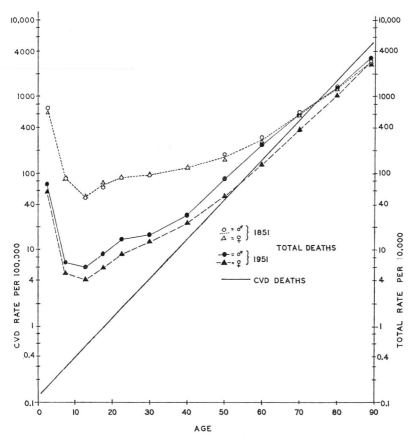

Fig. XII–2. Age and sex-specific annual mortality rates for all deaths in England (1851 and 1951) in cases per 10,000 population. Heavy line refers to CVD deaths in US-England (c. 1960) in cases per 100,000 population. English mortality data are in Appendix Table XII–a–2, from TAYLOR (1964)

hypertension and diabetes are obviously important in their own right, I could find no good evidence that their control alters the occurrence of stroke — at least of non-hemorrhagic stroke.

As physicians, we treat with all measures at hand the patient with carcinomatosis; as physicians too, we treat the stroke patient to the best of our ability. Certainly the intensive use of supportive care in the acute stages and of early and aggressive rehabilitation measures continuing thereafter to maximal benefit are vitally important in managing CVD. But I do think we might borrow a leaf from a different book: politics has been defined as the art of the possible. May this not be pertinent too in stroke ?

References

Aronson 18   TAYLOR 358   ZUMOFF 412
KOHN   181   World Health Organization 393

Chapter XIII

Summary by Chapters

Chapter I. Epidemiology is concerned with the occurrence, cause, and course of disease within populations, and the discovery of factors which tend to precipitate or prevent its appearance. Basic to this study is the definition of the disease, which is a necessary prerequisite to the determination of its frequency. The principal methods to ascertain the latter are the calculation of prevalence and incidence rates, and, for some disorders, mortality rates. The prevalence (rate) of a disease is the number of cases per unit population present at one time, and the incidence and mortality rates refer to the number of new cases or the number of deaths per unit population taking place in a given period, usually one year.

The major resources for epidemiologic study are hospital series, mortality statistics, and population surveys, the last being concerned with prevalence and incidence studies as well as with prospective long-term observations. All methods have assets and liabilities. The assets are diagnostic accuracy, detailed assessment, and some follow-up for hospital series, large numbers in time and space for mortality data, and completeness and representativeness for population surveys. The liabilities are input bias (selectivity) for hospital series, diagnostic inadequacy and selectivity for mortality data, and small numbers with few studies for population surveys.

Statistical testing of data is essential in the assessment of results, but most epidemiologic work does not permit the rigorous rejection of hypotheses after testing, because all the variables in "survey" material are neither controllable nor known. Calculation of confidence limits for frequency data and application of χ-square contingency tests are the major methods of use in epidemiologic studies. The latter is valuable in ascertaining deviations from homogeneous geographic distribution, which may well be of biologic import if the deviations are also large and are also patterned, i.e. forming clusters. Associations between distributions can be tested by calculating coefficients of correlation, and for epidemiologic data the non-parametric Spearman rank-order coefficient of correlation is often the procedure of choice.

Chapter II. The basic categorization of cerebrovascular disease is that of the International Statistical Classification of Diseases, Injuries, and Causes of Death, with the categories of subarachnoid hemorrhage (330), cerebral hemorrhage (331), cerebral thrombosis-embolism (332), and other and ill-defined vascular lesions affecting central nervous system (334). The rubric for cerebral artery spasm (333) is of little value.

Upon this base we can build clinical definitions. For subarachnoid hemorrhage (SAH), this includes those due to aneurysm, to arteriovenous malformation (AVM), to hypertension and/or arteriosclerosis, to miscellaneous diseases, and to no known disease ("idiopathic"). Sites of aneurysm and AVM are also noted. Cerebral hemorrhage needs no subdivisions.

Cerebral thrombosis-embolism is divisible into cerebral thrombosis, with its subunits of "thrombosis in evolution" and the "completed stroke"; transient ischemic attacks; cerebral embolism; and, in some works, "thorem" (*th*rombosis *or em*bolism). Anatomically one can consider each of these as involving the carotid system or the vertebrobasilar system from origin to end-arterioles; encephalomalacia can also be classified by location.

Chapter III. Validation of mortality data is an extremely complex matter. Correlation of such material with autopsy findings is subject to severe bias unless autopsy rates approach 100% of deaths, since it is generally the unusual or unknown for which post mortems are sought. In the United States, for cerebrovascular diseases as a whole, errors of omission as determined by autopsy material would seem to be some 10 to 15%, while errors of commission (over-reporting) some 10 to 40% of CVD deaths. These estimates are from major (white) population centers with high medical standards. In northern Europe, CVD deaths as a whole appear substantiated in some 75 to 100% and missed clinically in 0 to 10% of cases. Diagnostic customs would seem similar in the United States, England, and Norway. From clinical reviews of deaths in the United States, about 70 to 85% of CVD were considered probably correct. While mortality data for CVD as a whole then would seem sufficiently accurate for use in these lands, the subdivisions of CVD would appear incorrectly differentiated in some 30 to 80% of cases. There is also evidence that even at present hemorrhage (331) is used when the proper classification is other CVD (334).

Chapter IV. In considering CVD as a whole, mortality data indicate that in the 1950's CVD deaths occurred at an annual frequency of one case per 1000 population, with little variation among most of the countries with high medical and reporting standards. About $^3/_4$ of all stroke deaths occur in those age 70 or over, and strokes account for some 15% of deaths at present among those age 60 or more. Comparability of mortality statistics for CVD among various times and countries is most easily obtained by means of age-specific mortality rates. When these rates are plotted on a logarithmic scale against age, a straight line results which rises steeply. For the United States, England and Wales, Ireland, Norway, Sweden, Denmark, and Canada, by either sex, and for periods tested between 1933 and 1964, all these age-specific CVD mortality rates fit quite closely the same line. The same results are seen in a special mortality study in San Francisco designed for accuracy of diagnoses. Thus it would appear that CVD as a whole occurs equally in all these lands and periods, and in both sexes.

Incidence studies of the disease from Connecticut, Minnesota, Carlisle (England), Missouri, and English general practices, would suggest that the age-specific incidence rates for CVD are approximately twice the respective mortality rates up to age 74, and the two rates tend to merge above that age. This would imply a case-fatality rate of about 50% for strokes at these ages with a considerable increase in this rate among the oldest patients. Incidence studies dealing with only a segment of the age-spectrum also fit well the appropriate parts of the age-specific CVD experience in the more complete studies.

The sex ratios for CVD as a whole are very close to unity when using population-based sex-specific rates, whether mortality or incidence. Even the hospital series in general tend to be equal, or equally in excess or deficit, for males and females. Thus there is no support for the idea that stroke as a whole is a sex-related entity at any age-group.

Chapter V. The geographic distribution of CVD within individual countries is determined by calculation of mortality rates for each county separately and expressing the results as percentages of the national mean mortality rate. Because of the skew age-distribution of CVD deaths, the population age 60 and over was used as the denominator in these assessments. Statistical analysis with χ-square contingency tests of the null hypothesis of homogeneity was also done. With large numbers of cases, such as with strokes, this method is too sensitive to determine the biologic significance of non-homogeneity, and decisions on the nature of the geographic distribution of stroke were rather based on the degree of variation and the location of high frequency areas. Arbitrarily variation beyond 25% of the national mean (75 to 125%) for at least several units was required for "biologic significance". High frequency regions were further required to be patterned or form a cluster rather than being scattered through the land before an essential dependence of the disease on environmental factor(s) would be inferred.

Sweden was assessed for urban CVD deaths in 1933 and all CVD deaths in 1960. In the former, variation was wide with county rates ranging from 69% of the national mean to 189%. However the highest areas were quite scattered, and a "focus" could not be defined unless one so included the northern half of the country and a separate cluster in the south.

The distribution of CVD deaths in 1960 in Sweden was much more uniform, with the range of county rates being 69 to 130% of the mean. Again the highest areas were scattered, and the previous southern "focus" was now below the mean. Only two high areas at 126 and 130% exceeded our arbitrary limit of 125%.

The distribution of CVD deaths in Norway in 1946 was relatively uniform, with the range being 77 to 136% of the national mean. Only the one area (at 136%) was outside of 25% of the mean. The two highest rates found were at opposite ends of the country.

Denmark in 1950 was evaluated for "CVD" deaths, that is neurologic deaths of which 85% were strokes. Distribution here too was relatively even and the range of "CVD" mortality rates by county was 72 to 139% of the national mean rate. Only two counties exceeded 125% of the mean. The three highest counties were as separate from one another as possible in this land.

In 1960 the (true) CVD distribution of Denmark again showed a limited range at but 81 to 131% of the mean. Only two areas were outside of 25% of the mean, and they were both different from those found for 1950. Mapping both 1950 and 1960 distributions according to statistical levels for each area did not alter the impressions.

Age-specific distributions for CVD deaths in Denmark in 1961 were determined among nine regions of the country. CVD death rates for those ages 45 to 54, 55 to 64, and 65 to 74 were all homogeneous by χ-square test; only the 75 and over group (with 3300 cases) showed statistical significance, and the range here was but 78 to 127% of the mean. Individual regions classed as "significantly" high vs. their own mean were *never* the same in any two age groups.

Correlation of medical facilities with CVD deaths in Scandinavia revealed no significant linear associations in Norway or Denmark for physicians, specialists, hospitals, hospital beds, or hospital admissions, nor was population density related to CVD. The early and late Danish stroke distributions were also unrelated. In Sweden in 1933 there were significant negative correlations between urban CVD deaths and hospital beds or admissions, all physicians (but not urban physicians), and population density. This CVD distribution showed a moderate positive correlation with the 1960 CVD.

In Ireland the distribution of CVD deaths in 1951–1955 was one of moderate variation, the range being 55 to 165% of the mean, but only two areas exceeded 125% of the national mean. Rates were based on population age 35 and older, which may have a bearing on a somewhat wider range than in the other recent studies, as this base would less effectively counter variations in age-structure in the counties than the use of population 60 and older. Difference in distributions between the sexes was considerable, and, together with the small range for most of the regions, results here would seem in keeping with the Scandinavian findings.

In the United States in 1959–1961, the average annual age-adjusted CVD mortality rates for whites age 35 to 64 among 48 states varied minimally, with a range of 68 to 168% of the mean for males (four states only over 125% of the mean) and 77 to 135% of the mean for females (three states above 125% of the mean). Mapping by percentiles suggested a "focus" for males in the deep South, but little more than random distribution for females.

Similar mapping of physician distributions in the United States suggested an inverse relationship with CVD. Though there was no significant linear correlation (r = —0.2) between MD distribution and the resultant of four CVD distributions (male and female for two separate periods a decade apart), mapping of specific MD and male CVD rates by state did show a definitite inverse relationship. There were no high CVD areas where physician rates were above the mean, and variability was a characteristic where physicians were few. Most importantly, in *all* areas where CVD deaths exceeded 115% of the mean, physicians were represented at 80% or less of their national mean frequency. Similar findings, though somewhat less striking, were apparent for the Scandinavian distributions.

Therefore, the general conclusion is that the geographic distribution of CVD deaths as a whole within countries is essentially uniform, that clustering of high-rate areas is not a feature of CVD, and that regions of high-frequency CVD death reports are generally the areas of less adequate medical facilities.

There is nothing apparent in the geographic distribution of all CVD within these lands which suggests any notable relationship with environmental factors; variations with medical care would appear related to reporting adequacy.

Chapter VI. Relative frequencies for types of CVD based on mortality statistics vary widely in different lands and times. Cerebral hemorrhage deaths ranged from 14 cases per 100,000 in Belgium to 101 in Finland among average annual mortality rates for 18 countries considered to have adequate medical and reporting standards; all rates referred to the same 1951–1958 period and were age-standardized to the US population. The weighted mean of these 18 indicated some 3% of CVD deaths were SAH, 54% cerebral hemorrhage, 29% cerebral thrombosis-embolism, and 14% "other" CVD. More recent mortality data from Denmark indicated a higher proportion, or from England a lower proportion, for cerebral hemorrhage. The trend with time would seem to be toward a lower frequency reported for cerebral hemorrhage and — usually — "other" CVD, and an increase in thrombosis and possibly in SAH deaths.

Hospital series are too variable to provide useful data on CVD proportions by type. Population surveys should give us definitive information, but they too deviate considerably. However, the weighted mean of the frequencies in four population studies is the best available evidence on their proportions, and would indicate that SAH comprises some 12% of CVD cases, cerebral hemorrhage 16%, thrombosis-embolism 62%, and "other" CVD 10%, during the past decade. Annual incidence rates are probably close to the following: SAH, 20 cases per 100,000; Cb Hem 40; Cb thr-emb 120; and "other" 20; for a total of 200 CVD per 100,000 population.

With arbitrary case-fatality rates assigned to each of these frequencies, the observed *population* proportions listed might provide *mortality* proportions of 8% for SAH, 30% for hemorrhage, 50% for thrombosis, and 12% for "other" CVD deaths. England-Wales mortality rates in 1960 are indeed near these figures.

Subarachnoid hemorrhage has an age distribution far different from the remaining CVD, with a mean age at death in Denmark of 56, over 20 years below the rest. In England-Wales this is also found. Average annual age-specific mortality rates for SAH in Denmark rise from 0.2 per 100,000 in childhood to 2 by age 40, and thereafter more slowly to a peak of 6 by age 72, above which there may be some decline. Similar studies from the Netherlands do not differ significantly. There is generally found a slight female preponderance for SAH deaths.

Data on clinical subdivisions of SAH are taken mostly from the massive Cooperative Study recently reported, and compared with those of other series. Aneurysm accounts for half the SAH cases, AVM 6%, hypertension and/or arteriosclerosis 15%, miscellaneous 6%, and "idiopathic" SAH 22%.

The age distribution for SAH with aneurysm was essentially the same as for all SAH. Aneurysms do show considerable differences between the sexes for age at bleed (47 male vs. 56 female), frequency of the condition (M/F = 0.7), and location of aneurysm. While overall the internal carotid region aneurysms comprised half the cases and anterior cerebral $1/3$, the former were much less common than this in males and the latter much more common. Middle cerebral and posterior circuit aneurysms were equal in both sexes. For all lateralizing aneurysms (save anterior cerebral) there was a preponderance on the right side.

AVM with or without SAH were found in a much younger group averaging about age 38 in the Cooperative Study and 26 in a Mayo Clinic series. Presence of bleeding was not consistently related to age, there was no age difference by sex, and a slight male preponderance of cases was not remarkable.

SAH with hypertension occurred at older ages, the mean being 55. Those with arteriosclerosis were age 64 and both HT/AS age 60. Generally males were a bit more numerous in the vascular SAH.

Idiopathic SAH showed the same age distribution as all SAH, again with little difference between the sexes.

From the age-distributions and case-fatality rates of the various types of SAH, an attempt was made to extrapolate SAH incidence rates from the Danish age-specific mortality rates. Rates were then about equal at all ages after childhood, as was also found in a direct incidence study in Finland. In the latter, general incidence was 16 and mortality 7 to 8 per 100,000.

A diagram showing the interrelationships of cause and effect in SAH was also presented in an effort to tie together this information.

Chapter VII. While we have posited that cerebral hemorrhage should comprise some 30% of CVD deaths and thrombosis some 50%, the observed frequencies in published mortality data vary so widely that I believe it is unsafe to differentiate between the two on this basis. Be that as it may, age-specific mortality rates in Denmark for hemorrhage, thrombosis, and "other" CVD showed a similar straight-line logarithmic relationship with age, and at any age the rates were respectively in proportions of about 10:3:1. The median age at death was some 78 years in each category. There is no statistically significant basis for believing that cerebral hemorrhage cases or deaths occur at a younger age than thrombosis. Sex ratios in cerebral hemorrhage would appear to be unity. Swedish findings are similar, but with 10:5:4 proportions.

In cerebral thrombosis-embolism, age-specific incidence or mortality rates too rise in a logarithmic fashion with age. Thrombotic stroke in childhood is rare, and then is a result of non-arteriosclerotic disease-processes. Non-hemorrhagic stroke in young adults appears to be merely the usual tail expected in any frequency distribution, though hypertension and diabetes may be more common as associated factors in the young.

Autopsy studies indicate that cerebral arteriosclerosis is a universal finding in adults, and that the frequency of complicated lesions of same (hemorrhage, thrombosis, or calcium in the plaque) rises steeply with age, as does the frequency of encephalomalacia. Some 5% of unselected routine autopsies have evidence of recent encephalomalacia, and (in a separate series) the same proportion of intracranial occlusions. Thromboembolic occlusions in general are half in the carotid (equally intracranial and extracranial), $1/4$ in the middle cerebral, and $1/4$ in the posterior circuit. Recent thromboses are more common, but still equal, in the carotid. Recent emboli are 60% in the middle cerebral and 20% in the intracranial carotid arteries. There is not a good correlation between the presence or degree of intracranial or extracranial stenosis and the presence of cerebral infarcts. In 8 of 14 instances of total proximal carotid (11) or vertebral (3) artery occlusion, the patients had never shown evidence of focal *or* diffuse cerebral involvement. Conversely, in half the cases of recent encephalomalacia cited elsewhere a pertinent intracranial occlusion could be demonstrated at autopsy.

Clinical subdivisions of thromboembolic stroke are those by site and by cause. Age distributions of carotid vs. vertebrobasilar lesions were the same. In one cooperative study, 8% of thromboembolic strokes were TIA and 57% thrombosis (half "evolving"); "thorem" (thrombosis or embolism) was found in 27%, and embolism in 7%. Carotid system thromboses were about twice as common as vertebrobasilar, and for embolism some 90% were in the carotid tree. "Thorem" is not listed elsewhere as a distinct category. From a number of sources embolism would seem to comprise about 10% of thromboembolic CVD.

TIA may be the modern man's "cerebral artery spasm". Frequency of involvement in the carotid system was some 54% of TIA with a difference by sex, being 61% in males and 45% in females. Overall, TIA was reported twice as often in males as in females and this ratio was even greater than this for carotid involvement; in the vertebrobasilar tree the sex ratio was 1.4. There is no strong evidence that the frequency or duration of individual TIA attacks varies by site or sex.

From a number of sources it would appear that (TIA apart) there is little sex difference in the entirety or components of thromboembolic CVD, though there is *probably* a modest male excess in the younger years, but this would seem to be less than 1.3 males to 1.0 females.

Chapter VIII. It has been repeatedly stated that CVD, especially cerebral hemorrhage, is much more common in Negroes than whites in the USA, and that both are phenomenally high in Japan. All evidence to this point came from mortality statistics.

Negro age-specific mortality rates in the United States are indeed about twice those of the white until the oldest ages, and males are higher than females. This is also the case in Memphis and probably in Charleston, but not to the extent indicated by the author of the latter study. By state, the highest Negro rates were in the southeast and rates were usually closer to those of whites in the north and west. In a Missouri CVD population study, the CVD incidence rate for Negroes bases on but 24 cases was 4.1 per 1000, while the white rate was 2.5. Correction for population undercount would probably reduce the Negro rate to less than 3 per 1000. In Baltimore and Chicago surveys of illness, white and Negro CVD rates were the same. In an employed Los Angeles group, 2.5% of whites and 1.3% of Negroes had strokes in a 12 year period.

Two veterans hospital series indicated Negro to white ratios for CVD to be not dissimilar from general expectation. Strokes in young adults occurred in whites, Negroes, and Puerto Ricans to the same extent as they were otherwise represented in a New York hospital. In Detroit, 62.7% of CVD patients were Negro, as were 60.3% of patients with other neurologic disease.

Mortality rates in American Indians were the same as whites; moderately higher rates for Chinese Americans and Japanese Americans were based on about 10 cases or so in each age-sex group, and would appear unreliable.

Negroes generally exceed whites in mortality rate only for hemorrhage and "other" CVD. The former category is often incorrectly used in the United States for non-specific stroke. Thus even in the mortality data it is the poorly-defined CVD which provides the Negro excess.

I believe that the best explanation for high Negro CVD death rate reports would appear to be a scarcity of medical facilities. Further, population and hospital data provide some support for the statement that there is *no* excess of stroke in the Negro; certainly an increased rate must be considered not proven.

In South Africa, white CVD mortality rates were similar to US-England experience. Asian and Coloured rates, based on modest numbers of cases, were similar to the US Negro. Hospital death frequencies for CVD in Johannesburg with very small numbers were about equal in whites and Bantus, and possibly somewhat higher in Asian (Indian) and Coloured (mixed). Proof of racial differences here would seem insufficient.

In Japan, CVD has consistently been reported far in excess of western experience since at least 1900. Male rates have generally been notably greater than female. Even in 1962 some 28% of deaths in the elderly were CVD (vs. 15% in Scandinavia). In a recent population survey of Japan over $1/_3$ of deaths in those 40 and older were attributed to CVD, with autopsies in but 13% of all deaths. Cerebral hemorrhage was 90% of all CVD in 1950 and 71% in 1962. CVD rates were highest in the northern part of the main island. Major cities seemed to me to be low.

Evidence that Hawaiian Japanese have CVD mortality rates intermediate between Japan and the United States appears to be inadequate. Racial differentiations within Hawaii are hampered as well by admixture and small populations.

There has been a striking decline in the CVD hemorrhage/thrombosis ratio of death reports in Japan, from 29 to 1 in 1950 to 4 to 1 in 1962. The above population survey ratio was 2 to 1.

An ongoing adult population survey of Hisayama, Japan showed the following changes in four years: autopsy rates from 15% to 99%; CVD as per cent of all deaths from 32% to 17%; hemorrhage/thrombosis deaths (numbers) from 6/2 to 3/7.

A study of CVD in Hiroshima between 1958—1964 preselected with the use of autopsies which were accomplished in 85% of these deaths (and deaths were 70% of these CVD), showed a hemorrhage/thrombosis ratio of 0.4 for cases and for deaths. Of the original series in which CVD was listed as a cause of death, only 22% were confirmed at autopsy.

As part of the ABCC study in Japan, there were 201 autopsied cases in Hiroshima and Nagasaki between 1950—1962 in which CVD had been officially listed as cause of death. Of these, only 20 or *10%* were confirmed at autopsy.

I conclude therefore that an excess of cerebral hemorrhage is clearly, and of CVD as a whole probably, an artefact of diagnostic fashion in Japan, and that here too there is no evidence for racial predilection in CVD. The infrequency of autopsies may have prevented discovery of erroneous diagnoses in the past.

Chapter IX. The most important variable associated with the occurrence of CVD is age. Strokes in young adults may be looked upon as the normal tail of any frequency distribution.

Hypertension seems to be most common among the obese, the Negro and those with a familial history of same, but the disorder(s) appear to be decreasing in the United States. Hypertensive deaths are concentrated in the eastern half of this country from New York to the Carolinas and inland to Illinois—Arkansas—Louisiana. Treatment of malignant hypertension does reduce the frequency of complications thereof, about $1/_3$ of which tend to be CVD. Geographic distributions of CVD and hypertension deaths in general show little relationship. Among thrombotic CVD cases, hypertension is reported in approximately half. The frequency of hypertension in the general population of the same age however might not be far different from this rate, but a true relationship between the risk of stroke and hypertension does seem substantiated from population survey material. The late course of thrombotic CVD is unrelated to blood pressure levels. There is some evidence from Sweden that cerebral hemorrhage might be prevented by treating hypertension.

Coronary artery disease has a geographic distribution far different from that of CVD. In the United States ASHD deaths are concentrated on either coast, though within California their distribution is random. Major risk factors for CAD are hypertension, elevated cholesterol levels, obesity, diabetes, cigarette smoking, and EKG changes, according to several prospective studies. Insofar as prevalence surveys indicate, CAD seems to be about $1/3$ to $1/4$ as frequent in Japan as in the U.S., though the same precipitants are found, and in these works hypertension is equally common in both lands. Some racial differences in South Africa are apparent in lower rates among the Coloured and extremely low rates among the Bantu. Most workers agree that CAD and CVD behave much differently from an epidemiologic viewpoint. Even though they often coexist in the same individual and share common precipitants, they seem to be different disorders.

Cholesterol and lipid elevations in patients with CVD appear not well documented since findings vary from study to study. A low-order positive relationship between cigarette smoking and CVD deaths does seem to be present. There is some evidence for a genetic influence in CVD, a stronger one in hypertension, and none in CAD from a comparison of concordance rates in twins. In another study the parents of patients with strokes had died of CVD at a rate four times expectation. Obesity appears to bear no consistent relationship with CVD. Any association of CVD with soft water, or with rainfall or calcium levels in water, seems tenuous at best, and a similar conclusion is pertinent for air concentrations of cadmium. There does appear to be an occupational risk of an excessively high CVD death rate among lead workers with prolonged exposure.

Chapter X. Age-specific mortality rates for CVD indicate neither substantial increase nor decrease in deaths attributed to stroke during this century. Crude mortality rates of course have risen as longevity has increased. A modest decline in deaths under age 75 for CVD has been attributed by some to a concomitant decrease in hypertensive deaths; if real, this change would seem more a reflection of better diagnostic standards.

SAH death and attack rates in the Netherlands have been essentially stable in the last fifteen years, despite the author's contrary contention, and the age-specific death rates there are similar to those in Denmark.

Cerebral hemorrhage death rates have remained quite stable over time, though their proportion of CVD deaths, in England at least, has declined. While again some decrease in age-specific death rates has been posited, this seems much more likely to be on the basis of changing diagnostic fashions than on a change in frequency. An English study which shows an excellent agreement in the ratios of hemorrhage to thrombosis deaths over time between an autopsy series and general mortality statistics could also be explained by a variety of sources of bias, which are considered in some detail; among these, the more recent hospital cases of thrombosis in that series would be inflated by increased bed utilization, especially for chronic care, and a consequent increase in autopsies for those dying with cerebral infarcts and not necessarily because of same.

Deaths attributed to cerebral thrombosis as noted have risen with time according to all available mortality data. In part this too must be regarded as a result of coding and diagnostic fashions, since both "other CVD" and cerebral hemorrhage together vary inversely as thrombosis. The extent of the increase though *seems* too great for this explanation, and we might therefore accept a "real" increase in Cb. thrombosis death certifications. However, it is still feasible to explain even the "real" increase on better diagnosis, with the retrieval in this category of a greater proportion of late deaths. Therefore a true increase in fatal cerebral thrombosis I believe also remains unproven.

Since population surveys for CVD are too recent and hospital series too biased, we have no data on changes in disease-frequency (rather than death-frequency) with time for either the parts or the whole of CVD (331 to 334), and therefore also can give no estimate of any possible changes in case-fatality rates. However, an *estimate* of relative proportions of CVD types to be expected at present in mortality data, based upon observed frequencies in population surveys and on case-fatality rates, provides proportions for all subdivisions of CVD which are close to the actual proportions found in England-Wales for 1960, including a thrombosis/hemorrhage ratio of 1.7.

It is probable that there has been no major change in the frequency of CVD deaths in this century. Whether there has been a true decline in cerebral hemorrhage and a concomitant increase in cerebral thrombosis warrants at best the Scottish verdict of "not proven".

Chapter XI. Here the evaluation of the course of CVD is limited to survival as demonstrated by cumulative case-fatality rates over time. The principal resources are (hospitalized) survivors of the ictus, hospital surveys, and the single population survey of Middlesex, Connecticut.

In considering all CVD together, survivors of the ictus had case-fatality rates of some 20% in six months and 60% in five years. Hospital series indicate 1 in 3 die in two months and half in two years. The population survey showed case-fatality rates to be much higher: half the patients were dead in two weeks and $^3/_4$ in one year; by five years 85% had expired. These patients were aged 74 at ictus, considerably older than those of the hospital series, and there was a striking correlation within the population study between case-fatality rate and age. Similar changes with age were noted in the hospital series. Thus the outcome (in terms of survival) is in very large measure a function of age at the time of the stroke.

For SAH, the Cooperative Aneurysm Study provides the most definitive information on course. Overall the cumulative fatality rates in the first three months after the bleed are 60% for single or multiple aneurysms, 22% for AVM, and 36% for all other SAH. Within this last group, SAH with hypertension had a fatality rate of 51%, SAH with arteriosclerosis 72%, and SAH with both HT and AS, 92%. "Idiopathic" SAH case fatality rate was 18%. Of considerable interest was the association of SAH fatalities with intracerebral hemorrhage: regardless of etiology some 80 to 90% of fatal cases had intraparenchymal hemorrhage, while its frequency in survivors was 0 to 24%. Acute deaths with aneurysm were more common than expected in those of the middle cerebral artery and less in those of the internal carotid region, probably because of the difference in associated intraparenchymal bleeding.

For cerebral hemorrhage the major source of information is the Middlesex population survey. Case-fatality rates in this elderly group were 59% in one week, 75% in two weeks, and 82% in one month. By five years 97% were dead. The time of death is much different from that for the cerebral thrombosis deaths in the same study, although the five-year survival rates do not differ significantly.

With cerebral thrombosis, survivors of the ictus had a low fatality rate in the first year, but about half were dead in five. The hospital series indicate one in four patients was dead in six months and one in three in two years, with $^1/_2$ to $^2/_3$ dead by five years. In the population survey (of older patients), one in three died early, $^1/_2$ were dead in six months and $^2/_3$ by one year; 84% had expired in five years. Differences between these results and those of the hospital series are explicable on the basis of age at ictus. Carotid system and basilar-vertebral strokes showed the same course.

Treatment series in thrombosis and TIA are cited but not discussed, although some arbitrary judgements on the value of various modalities are offered.

Chapter XII. In an attempt to tie together the work presented here, some strictly personal opinions are offered. We may begin by suggesting some revisions of the ISC coding of CVD diseases and deaths. First, I would remove SAH and hypertensive encephalopathy from the group, assigning a new category for SAH, and putting all hypertensive encephalopathy under malignant hypertension (code 445). With the differences in cause, age, and behavior, I see no reason why SAH should be included in "stroke". Second, remove all ambiguities from the code for cerebral hemorrhage so that no condition other than cerebral hemorrhage is included. Third, delete cerebral artery spasm.

The proposed new coding, each one mutually exclusive, would be as follows: cerebral hemorrhage (331); cerebral thrombosis, with all its equivalents (332); cerebral embolism (333); transient ischemic attacks (334); spinal thrombosis and hemorrhage (335); cerebral arteriosclerosis, general (336); cerebral venous thrombosis, non-pyogenic, which includes venous sinuses (337); CVD, not elsewhere classified (338). Total CVD (331—338). The new code suggested for SAH would be: SAH with aneurysm (358); SAH, other non-traumatic (359).

Residua of stroke should be classed with CVD, whether in morbidity or mortality statistics. One way would be the use of subcoding, as 331.1 for "residua of cerebral hemorrhage".

The geographic distribution of CVD as a whole both within and among nations is such that the disorder seems essentially uniform with no suggestion of its dependence on exogenous factors.

From international mortality comparisons and clinical data a similar conclusion seems warranted for SAH. Mortality data can *not* I believe be separated with any degree of assurance, but with a posited "true" frequency of some $^1/_3$ of all CVD deaths as hemorrhage and almost all the rest as thrombosis, mortality data for the whole would seem to be referable also to either entity, unless one posits a reciprocal relationship between the two. Therefore we can conclude cerebral hemorrhage and thromboembolic stroke also demonstrate no evidence of dependence on exogenous factors. Clinical and population data of widely varied geographic sources would tend to support this conclusion.

In general, sex ratios in CVD in whole or in part are essentially unity. The only exceptions are a *possible* male excess in young non-hemorrhagic stroke, a 2-to-1 male preponderance reported in TIA, and a female excess (1.4 to 1) in aneurysmal SAH, with other oddities in this last (older age in women, even more of a female excess in internal carotid aneurysms).

The racial characteristics of CVD are fascinating. The available evidence indicates (to me) that there is *no* excess of cerebral hemorrhage or CVD in the US Negro *or* in Japan. In fact, one might predict that areas or groups cited as having high frequencies will be found to show a scarcity of medical facilities in numbers or utilization. In Japan however, the major reason must be diagnostic customs and tradition coupled with low autopsy rates.

Associated factors of importance in CVD (excluding SAH) would of course be hypertension in hemorrhage, and for thromboembolic stroke, low-order relationships with hypertension, smoking, and diabetes. The high prevalence of hypertension and CAD in the population at risk for stroke makes their specificity much less tenable and the associations themselves much less meaningful. Constituents of blood lipids and drinking water would not appear well documented as related variables. Limited evidence does however suggest that genetic factors play a role in CVD.

Again excluding SAH, the most dramatic factor in CVD is its relationship with age, which is one of a logarithmic increase. Frequency of intravascular occlusions and of encephalomalacia also rise with age as do autopsies in general. Comparison of age-specific mortality rates for all deaths in England and Wales between 1851 and 1951 shows a very similar curve above age 55 at both periods. Superimposing these on the US-England CVD mortality rates brings out the marked similarity in the curves between all recent adult deaths and CVD deaths. We might hypothesize that as we remove treatable deaths, the age-specific mortality curve of the population will reach that which is intrinsic to the human aging-process (whatever is included in that term). The CVD mortality curve appears to describe such a line. If this be correct, then stroke may have to be classed as a concomitant of aging, and as such would seem to be preventable only to the extent that one could reverse the aging process.

References

(asterisks refer to general monographs)

1. ACHESON, J., and E. C. HUTCHINSON: Observations on the natural history of transient cerebral ischaemia. Lancet **1964 II**, 871—874.
2. ACHESON, R. M.: Mortality from cerebrovascular accidents and hypertension in the Republic of Ireland. Brit. J. prev. soc. Med. **14**, 139—147 (1960).
3. — The etiology of coronary heart disease: a review from the epidemiological standpoint. Yale J. Biol. Med. **35**, 143—170 (1962).
4. — The epidemiology of stroke. Lancet **1964 I**, 494—495.
5. — (1) Mortality from cerebrovascular disease in the United States. Publ. Hlth. Monogr. **76**, 23—40 (1966).
6. — (2) Personal communication, Yale University, June 8, (1966).
7. ADAMS, G. F.: Prospects for patients with strokes, with special reference to the hypertensive hemiplegic. Brit. med. J. **1965 II**, 253—259.
8. —, and J. D. MERRETT: Prognosis and survival in the aftermath of hemiplegia. Brit. med. J. **1967 I**, 309—314.
9. ad hoc Committee, Advisory Council for the National Institute of Neurological Diseases and Blindness, Public Health Service: A classification and outline of cerebrovascular diseases. Neurology (Minneap.) 8, (part 2) 1—34 (1958).
10. ADIN, B.: Personal communications, National Board of Health of Sweden, June 15 and July 20, 1964.
11. AF BJÖRKESTEN, G., and V. HALONEN: Incidence of intracranial vascular lesions in patients with subarachnoid hemorrhage investigated by four-vessel angiography. J. Neurosurg. **23**, 29—32 (1965).
12. —, and H. TROUPP: Prognosis of subarachnoid hemorrhage: a comparison between patients with verified aneurysms and patients with normal angiograms. J. Neurosurg. **14**, 434—441 (1957).
13. AHMED, R. H., and C. B. SEDZIMIR: Ruptured anterior communicating aneurysm. A comparison of medical and specific surgical treatment. J. Neurosurg. **26**, 213—217 (1967).
14. den Almindelige Danske Laegeforening: Laegeforeningens Aarborg 1950—1951: 33te Aargang, Afd. II, København 1950.
15. ALSING, I.: Personal communications, National Health Service of Denmark, April 22, June 6, July 30, 1964.
16. — Personal communication, Sept. 9, 1966.
17. ARKIN, H., and R. R. COLTON: Tables for Statisticians. Second Ed. New York: Barnes and Noble 1963.
18. ARONSON, S. M., and B. E. ARONSON: Ischemic cerebral vascular disease. Frequency in autopsy population. N. Y. St. J. Med. **66**, 954—957 (1966).
19. ARSENI, C., S. IONESCU, M. MARETSIS, and M. GHITESCU: Primary intraparenchymatous hematomas. J. Neurosurg. **27**, 207—215 (1967).
20. ASK-UPMARK, E., and D. INGVAR: A follow-up examination of 138 cases of subarachnoid hemorrhage. Acta med. scand. **138**, 15—31 (1950).
21. AURELL, M., and B. HOOD: Cerebral hemorrhage in a population after a decade of active antihypertensive treatment. Acta med. scand. **176**, 377—383 (1964).
22. BAKER, R. N.: An evaluation of anticoagulant therapy in the treatment of cerebrovascular disease. Report of the Veterans Administration Cooperative Study of Atherosclerosis, Neurology Section. Neurology (Minneap.) 11 (part 2), 132—138 (1961).
23. — (1) Anticoagulants in the prevention and management of strokes. In: DEFOREST, R. E. (ed): Proceedings of the National Stroke Congress, pp. 50—57. Springfield, Ill.: Charles C Thomas 1966.

24. BAKER, R. N.: Anticoagulant therapy in cerebral infarction. Report on cooperative study. Neurology 12, 823—835 (1962).

25. —, W. S. SCHWARTZ, and A. S. ROSE: (2) Transient ischemic strokes. A report of a study of anticoagulant therapy. Neurology 16, 841—847 (1966).

26. BALOW, J., M. ALTER, and J. A. RESCH: Cerebral thromboembolism. A clinical appraisal of 100 cases. Neurology 16, 559—564 (1966).

27. BATTACHARJI, S. K., E. C. HUTCHINSON, and A. J. McCALL: Stenosis and occlusion of vessels in cerebral infarction. Brit. med. J. 1967 3, 270—274.

28. BEHREND, R.-C.: Eine neue neurologische Wissenschaft, die „Geoneurologie" Mitt. Max-Planck-Gesell. 3, 144—154 (1963).

29. BENNETT, C. G., G. H. TOKUYAMA, and T. C. McBRIDE: Cardiovascular-renal mortality in Hawaii. Amer. J. publ. Hlth. 52, 1418—1431 (1962).

30. BERKSON, D. M., and J. STAMLER: Epidemiological findings on cerebrovascular diseases and their implications. J. Atheroscler. Res. 5, 189—202 (1965).

31. BIANCONE, S.: L'età dei morti per malattie cardiovascolari in Italia (medie dei trienni 1953—1955 e 1959—1961). Ann. Sanità pubbl. 25, 808—827 (1964).

32. BICKERSTAFF, E. R., and J. MacD. HOLMES: Cerebral arterial insufficiency and oral contraceptives. Brit. Med. J. 1967 I, 726—729.

33. BIÖRCK, G.: Course and prognosis in some cardiac diseases. J. chron. Dis. 15, 9—28 (1962).

34. —, H. BOSTRÖM, and A. WIDSTRÖM: On the relationship between water hardness and death rates in cardiovascular diseases. Acta med. scand. 178, 239—252 (1965).

35. BLAKEMORE, W. S., W. H. HARDESTY, J. E. BEVILACQUA, and T. A. TRISTAN: Reversal of blood flow in the right vertebral artery accompanying occlusion of the innominate artery. Ann. Surg. 161, 353—356 (1965).

36. BORHANI, N. O.: (1) Changes and geographic distribution of mortality from cerebrovascular disease. Amer. J. Publ. Hlth 55, 673—681 (1965).

37. — (2) Magnitude of the problem of cardiovascular-renal diseases, in the President's Commision: Report to the President. A National Program to Conquer Heart Disease, Cancer, and Stroke, Volume II, pp. 14—47. Washington, D. C.: U. S. Govt. Printing Office 1965.

38. —, H. H. HECHTER, and L. BRESLOW: Report of a ten-year follow-up study of the San Francisco longshoremen: Mortality from coronary heart disease and from all causes. J. chron. Dis. 16, 1251—1266 (1963).

39. BOYLE, R. W., and M. REID: What happens to the stroke victim. Geriatrics 20, 949—955 (1965).

40. BRADSHAW, P., and P. McQUAID: The syndrome of vertebro-basilar insufficiency. Quart. J. Med. 32, 279—296 (1963).

41. BREWIS, M., D. C. POSKANZER, C. ROLLAND, and H. MILLER: Neurological disease in an English city. Acta neurol. scand. 42, suppl. 24, 1—89 (1966).

42. BRYANT, L. R., B. EISEMAN, F. C. SPENCER, and A. LIEBER: Frequency of extracranial cerebrovascular disease in patients with chronic psychosis. New Engl. J. Med. 272, 12—17 (1965).

43. —, and F. C. SPENCER: Occlusive disease of subclavian artery. J. Amer. med. Ass. 196, 123—128 (1966).

44. BULL, J. W. D.: Contribution of radiology to the study of intracranial aneurysms. Brit. med. J. 1962 II, 1701—1708.

45. Bureau de la Statistique Générale, Cabinet Impérial: Etat de la Population de L'Empire du Japon au 31 Décembre 1913, Tokio 1916.

46. — Résumé Statistique de L'Empire du Japon. 28° Année, Tokio 1914.

47. — Statistique des Causes de Décès de L'Empire du Japon pendant l'An XLIII de Meiji 1910. Tome I (Fu, Ken, et Hokkaido ou Districts), Tokio 1913.

48. Bureau of the Census, U.S. Dept. of Commerce: Manual of the International List of Causes of Death as Adopted for Use in the United States. Washington, D. C.: U.S. Govt. Printing Office 1940.

49. BURGESS, A. M., JR., T. COLTON, and O. L. PETERSON: Categorical programs for heart disease, cancer, and stroke. Lessons from international death-rate comparisons. New Engl. J. Med. 273, 533—537 (1965).

50. BURROWS, E. H., and J. MARSHALL: Angiographic investigation of patients with transient ischaemic attacks. J. Neurol. Neurosurg. Psychiat. **28**, 533—539 (1965).

51. CARROLL, D.: The disability in hemiplegia caused by cerebrovascular disease: serial studies of 98 cases. J. chron. Dis. **15**, 179—188 (1962).

52. CARROLL, R. E.: The relationship of cadmium in the air on cardiovascular disease death rates. J. Amer. med. Ass. **198**, 267—269 (1966).

53. CARTER, A. B.: Ingravescent cerebral infarction. Quart. J. Med. **29**, 611—625 (1960).

54. — Strokes: natural history and prognosis. Proc. roy. Soc. Med. **56**, 483—486 (1963).

55. Central Statistics Office: Tuarascáil an Ard-Chláraitheora 1951, Stationery Office, Dublin 1955.

56. CHAPMAN, J. M., L. G. REEDER, and E. R. BORUN: Epidemiology of vascular lesions affecting the central nervous system: the occurrence of strokes in a sample population under observation for cardiovascular disease. Amer. J. publ. Hlth. **56**, 191—201 (1966).

57. CLEMMENSEN, J.: Statistical studies in the aetiology of malignant neoplasms. I. Review and results. II. Basic tables. Denmark 1943—1957. København: Munksgaard 1965, 1964.

58. CODER, D. M., R. L. FRYE, P. E. BERNATZ, and S. G. SHEPS: Symptomatic bilateral "subclavian steal". Proc. Mayo Clin. **40**, 473—476 (1965).

59. COLE, M.: Strokes in young women using oral contraceptives. Arch. intern. Med. **120**, 551—555 (1967).

60. Commission on Chronic Illness: Chronic Illness in the United States. Volume IV. Chronic Illness in a Large City. The Baltimore Study. Cambridge, Mass.: Harvard Univ. Press 1957.

61. CONANT, R. G., J. A. PERKINS, and A. B. AINLEY: Stroke morbidity, mortality and rehabilitative potential. J. chron. Dis. **18**, 397—403 (1965).

62. CONNOR, W. E.: Dietary cholesterol and the pathogenesis of atherosclerosis. Geriatrics **16**, 407—415 (1961).

63. COOK, A. W., D. M. DOOLEY, and E. J. BROWDER: Anterior communicating aneurysms: treatment by ligation of an anterior cerebral artery. J. Neurosurg. **23**, 371—374 (1965).

64. CRAWFORD, M. D., and M. SARNER: Ruptured intracranial aneurysm. Community study. Lancet **1965 II**, 1254—1257.

65. CROFTON, E., and J. CROFTON: Influence of smoking on mortality from various diseases in Scotland and in England and Wales. An analysis by cohorts. Brit. med. J. **1963 II**, 1161—1164.

66. CROMPTON, M. R.: The pathology of ruptured middle-cerebral aneurysms with special reference to the differences between the sexes. Lancet **1962 II**, 421—423.

67. — Mechanism of growth and rupture in cerebral berry aneurysms. Brit. med. J. **1966 I**, 1138—1142.

68. CUMINGS, J. N., I. K. GRUNDT, J. T. HOLLAND, and J. MARSHALL: Serum-lipids and cerebrovascular disease. Lancet **1967 II**, 194—195.

69. DALAL, P. M.: Incidence of cerebral vascular lesions at the Nair Hospital, Bombay. Neurology of India (Bombay) **13**, 37—39 (1965).

70. DALSGAARD-NIELSEN, T.: Survey of 1000 cases of apoplexia cerebri. Acta psychiat. neurol. scand. **30**, 169—185 (1955).

71. DAVID, N. J., and A. HEYMAN: Factors influencing the prognosis of cerebral thrombosis and infarction due to atherosclerosis. J. chron. Dis. **11**, 394—404 (1960).

72. DAVIE, J. C., and W. COXE: Occlusive disease of the carotid artery in children. Carotid thrombectomy with recovery in a 2-year-old boy. Arch. Neurol. (Chic.) **17**, 313—323 (1967).

73. DAWBER, T. R., W. B. KANNEL, P. M. McNAMARA, and M. E. COHEN: An epidemiologic study of apoplexy ("strokes"). Observations in 5,209 adults in the Framingham study on association of various factors in the development of apoplexy. Trans. Amer. neurol. Ass. **90**, 237—240 (1965).

74. — —, N. REVOTSKIE, and A. KAGAN: The epidemiology of coronary heart disease: the Framingham inquiry. Proc. roy. Soc. Med. **55**, 265—271 (1962).

75. — — —, J. STOKES III, A. KAGAN, and T. GORDON: Some factors associated with the development of coronary heart disease; six years follow-up experience with the Framingham study. Amer. J. publ. Hlth. **49**, 1349—1356 (1959).

76. DeBakey, M. E.: The surgical approach to strokes. Postgrad. Med. **39**, 343—348 (1966).
77.* DeForest, R. E. (Ed.): Proceedings of the National Stroke Congress. Rehabilitation-Management-Prevention. Springfield, Ill.: Charles C Thomas 1966.
78. Diamond, E. L., and A. M. Lilienfeld: Effects of errors in classification and diagnosis in various types of epidemiological studies. Amer. J. publ. Hlth. **52**, 1137—1144 (1962).
79. — — Misclassification errors in 2×2 tables with one margin fixed: some further comments. Amer. J. publ. Hlth. **52**, 1206—1210 (1962).
80. Dingwall-Fordyce, I., and R. E. Lane: A follow-up study of lead workers. Brit. J. industr. Med. **20**, 313—315 (1963).
81. Division of Health and Welfare Statistics, Welfare Minister's Secretariat, Japan: Vital Statistics 1950, Parts II—IV, Part I, Tokyo (1952, 1953).
82. Doll, R. (Ed.): Methods of Geographical Pathology; Report of the Study Group Convened by the Council, Council for International Organizations of Medical Sciences. Springfield, Ill.: Charles C Thomas 1959.
83. —, and A. B. Hill: Mortality of British doctors in relation to smoking: observations on coronary thrombosis. Nat. Cancer Inst. Monogr. **19**, 205—268 (1966).
84. Dorndorf, W.: Gegenwärtiger Stand der chirurgischen Behandlung des cerebrovasculären Insultes. Nervenarzt **36**, 18—30 (1965).
85. Dreyer, K., E. Frandsen, and H. Hamtoft: Medicostatistical information from Denmark for the years 1960 and 1961. Dan. med. Bull. **10**, 26—32 (1963).
86. — — — Medicostatistical information from Denmark for the years 1961 and 1962. Dan. med. Bull. **11**, 98—104 (1964).
87. du Boulay, G. H.: Some observations on the natural history of intracranial aneurysms. Brit. J. Radiol. **38**, 721—757 (1965).
88.* Duckert, F., and F. Streuli (Ed.): Pathogenesis and treatment of thromboembolic diseases, including coronary, cerebral and peripheral thrombosis. Stuttgart: F. K. Schattauer-Verlag 1966.
89. Dunsmore, R. H., and J. L. Polcyn: Subarachnoid hemorrhage: prognostic factors. J. Neurosurg. **13**, 165—169 (1956).
90. Dustan, H. P., R. E. Schneckloth, A. C. Corcoran, and I. H. Page: The effectiveness of long-term treatment of malignant hypertension. Circulation **18**, 644—651 (1958).
91. Editorial: Recurrent cerebral ischaemia. Lancet **1964 II**, 799—800.
92. Editorial: Blood pressure and age. Brit. med. J. **1967 II**, 650—651.
93. Eisenberg, H., J. T. Morrison, P. Sullivan, and F. M. Foote: Cerebrovascular accidents. Incidence and survival rates in a defined population, Middlesex County, Connecticut. J. Amer. med. Ass. **189**, 883—888 (1964).
94.* Engel, A., and T. Larsson: Thule International Symposia. Stroke. Symposium 19.—21. April 1966. Stockholm: Nord. Bokh. Förlag 1967.
95. Enger, E., and S. Bøyesen: Long-term anticoagulant therapy in patients with cerebral infarction. A controlled clinical study. Acta med. scand. **178**, suppl. 438, 1—61 (1965).
96. Erhardt, C. L., L. Weiner, and G. McAvoy: Pathological reports for mortality statistics. J. Amer. med. Ass. **171**, 33—36 (1959).
97. Ericson, H. L.: The epidemiology and treatment of strokes in Lake County, Illinois. Illinois med. J. **128**, 338—343 (1965).
98. Fearnley, G. R., R. Chakrabarti, E. Hocking, and J. F. Evans: Fibrinolytic effects of diguanides plus ethyloestrenol in occlusive vascular disease. Lancet **1967 II**, 1008 to 1011.
99. Fejfar, Z., D. Badger, and M. Grais: Epidemiological aspects of thrombosis and vascular disease. In: Duckert, F., and F. Streuli (Ed.), Pathogenesis and treatment of thromboembolic diseases, pp. 5—19 (1966).
100. Feldman, R. G., and M. J. Albrink: Serum lipids and cerebrovascular disease. Arch. Neurol. (Chic.) **10**, 91—100 (1964).
101. Felger, G. P., H. Reisner und E. Scherzer: Das weitere Schicksal von 1000 zerebralen Insulten. Wien. klin. Wschr. **73**, 397—402 (1961).
102.* Fields, W. S. (Ed.): Pathogenesis and treatment of cerebrovascular disease. Springfield, Ill.: Charles C Thomas 1961.

103.* —, and W. A. SPENCER: Stroke rehabilitation: basic concepts and research trends. St. Louis, Mo.: W. H. Green, Inc. 1967.

104. FISHER, C. M.: (1) Anticoagulant therapy in cerebral thrombosis and cerebral embolism: a national cooperative study, interim report. Neurology (Minneap.) 11 (part 2), 119—131 (1961).

105. — (2) The pathology and pathogenesis of intracerebral hemorrhage. In: W. S. FIELDS, Pathogenesis and treatment of cerebrovascular disease, pp. 295—317. Springfield, Ill.: Charles C Thomas 1961.

106. —, I. GORE, N. OKABE, and P. D. WHITE: Atherosclerosis of the carotid and vertebral arteries — extracranial and intracranial. J. Neuropath. exp. Neurol. 24, 455—476 (1965).

107. FISHER, R. A.: Statistical methods for research workers. 13. Ed.-revised. New York: Hafner Publ. Co. 1958.

108. — Statistical methods and scientific inference. 2. Ed., revised. New York: Hafner Publ. Co. 1959.

109. —, and F. YATES: Statistical tables for biological, agricultural, and medical research. 6. Ed., revised and enlarged. New York: Hafner Publ. Co. 1963.

110. FISHER, R. G., and E. SACHS, JR.: Carotid artery surgery for cerebrovascular accident. Geriatrics 16, 508—514 (1961).

111. FLETCHER, C. M., and P. D. OLDHAM: Prevalence surveys. In: L. J. WITTS, Medical surveys and clinical trials, 2nd ed., pp. 50—70. London: Oxford Univ. Press 1964.

112. FLOREY, C. DUV., M. SENTER, and R. M. ACHESON: A study of the validity of the diagnosis of stroke in mortality data. I. Certificate analysis. Yale J. Biol. Med. 40, 148—163 (1967).

113. FOLGER, G. M., and K. D. SHAH: Subclavian steal in patients with Blalock-Taussig anastomosis. Circulation 31, 241—248 (1965).

114. FORD, A. B., and S. KATZ: Prognosis after strokes. Part I. A critical review. Medicine (Baltimore) 45, 223—236 (1966).

115. FRANCIS, T., JR.: The epidemiological approach to human ecology. Amer. J. med. Sci. 237, 667—684 (1959).

116. FUMAGALLI, C., F. PAPINI, e V. ZUCCONI: Indagine statistica sulla mortalità per vasculopatie cerebrali. G. Geront. 12, 1057—1069 (1964).

117. GEIGER, H. J., and N. A. SCOTCH: The epidemiology of essential hypertension. A review with special attention to psychologic and sociocultural factors. I: Biologic mechanisms and descriptive epidemiology. J. chron. Dis. 16, 1151—1182 (1963).

118. General Register Office: The Registrar General's Statistical Review of England and Wales for the Year 1960, Part I, Tables, Medical. London: H. M. Stationery Office 1962.

119. GERMAN, W. J., and S. P. W. BLACK: Cervical ligation for internal carotid aneurysms. An extended follow-up. J. Neurosurg. 23, 572—577 (1965).

120. GIBBS, J. R.: Effects of carotid ligation on the size of internal carotid aneurysms. J. Neurol. Neurosurg. Psychiat. 28, 383—394 (1965).

121. GIEL, R.: Notes on the epidemiology of spontaneous subarachnoid haemorrhages. Psychiat. Neurol. Neurochir. 68, 265—271 (1965).

122. GIFFORD, A. J.: An epidemiological study of cerebrovascular disease. Amer. J. Publ. Hlth 56, 452—461 (1966).

123. GIFFORD, R. W., JR.: Hypertensive cardiovascular disease. Effect of antipressor therapy on the course and prognosis. Amer. J. Cardiol. 17, 656—662 (1966).

124. GILROY, J., and J. S. MEYER: Auscultation of the neck in occlusive cerebrovascular disease. Circulation 25, 300—310 (1962).

125.* GOLDBERG, I. D., and L. T. KURLAND: Mortality in 33 countries from diseases of the nervous system. Wld. Neurol. 3, 444—465 (1962).

126.* GOLDSCHMIDT, E. (Ed.): The genetics of migrant and isolate populations. Baltimore: Williams and Wilkins Co. 1963.

127. GORDON, E. E., E. BRECKINRIDGE, W. GELLMAN, and H. MACKLER: Stroke-community services. Nat. Conf. Cardiovasc. Dis. 2, 761—777 (1964).

128. GORDON, P. C.: The epidemiology of cerebral vascular disease in Canada: an analysis of mortality data. Canad. med. Ass. J. 95, 1004—1011 (1966).

129. GORDON, T.: Mortality experience among the Japanese in the United States, Hawaii, and Japan. Publ. Hlth Rep. (Wash.) **72**, 543—553 (1957).
130. GRIFFITH, G. W., and G. A. V. MORGAN: Diagnostic precision as a factor in male mortality data. Brit. J. prev. soc. Med. **15**, 68—78 (1961).
131. GROCH, S. N.: (1) Discussion on anticoagulant therapy. Neurology (Minneap.) **11**, (part 2) 141—144 (1961).
132. —, E. McDEVITT, and I. S. WRIGHT: (2) A long-term study of cerebral vascular disease. Ann. intern. Med. **55**, 358—367 (1961).
133. GURDJIAN, E. S., W. R. DARMODY, D. W. LINDNER, and L. M. THOMAS: The fate of patients with carotid and vertebral artery surgery for stenosis or occlusion. Surg. Gynec. Obstet. **121**, 326—330 (1965).
134. —, W. G. HARDY, D. W. LINDNER, and L. M. THOMAS: (1) Analysis of occlusive disease of the carotid artery and the stroke syndrome. J. Amer. med. Ass. **176**, 194—204 (1961).
135. —, D. W. LINDNER, W. G. HARDY, and L. M. THOMAS: (2) Incidence of surgically treatable lesions in cases studied angiographically. Neurology (Minneap.) **11**, (part 2) 150—152 (1961).
136. —, and L. M. THOMAS: Evaluation and indications for surgery in extracranial cerebro-vascular disease. J. Neurosurg. **26**, 235—243 (1967).
137.* HAENSZEL, W.: Epidemiological approaches to the study of cancer and other chronic diseases. Nat. Cancer Inst. Monogr. **19**, U.S.P.H.S. Bethseda, Md.: U.S. Govt. Printing Office 1966.
138. HAMBY, W. B.: Intracranial aneurysms. Springfield, Ill.: Charles C Thomas 1952.
139. HAMILTON, M., E. N. THOMPSON, and T. K. M. WISNIEWSKI: The role of blood-pressure control in preventing complications of hypertension. Lancet **1964 I**, 235—238.
140. HAMMOND, E. C.: Smoking in relation to mortality and morbidity. Findings in first thirty-four months of follow-up in a prospective study started in 1959. J. nat. Cancer Inst. **32**, 1161—1188 (1964).
141. — Smoking in relation to the death rates of one million men and women. Nat. Cancer Inst. Monogr. **19**, 127—204 (1966).
142. HAMTOFT, H., and J. MOSBECH: Om primaere og sekundaere dødsårsager. Ugeskr. Laeg. **123**, 1363—1364 (1961).
143. HARDIN, C. A.: Operative treatment of multiple sites of extracranial cervical artery occlusions. Circulation **33/34**, suppl. 1, I-173—I-176 (1966).
144. HARINGTON, M., P. KINCAID-SMITH, and J. McMICHAEL: Results of treatment in malignant hypertension. A seven-year experience in 94 cases. Brit. med. J. **1959 II**, 969—980.
145. HARVALD, B., and M. HAUGE: Hereditary factors elucidated by twin studies. In: NEEL, J. V., M. W. SHAW, and W. J. SCHULL: Genetics and the epidemiology of chronic diseases, pp. 61—76. Washington: P.H.S., Publ. No. 1163, 1965.
146. Health and welfare statistics division, Minister's secretariat, Ministry of Health and Welfare: Vital Statistics 1962, Japan, Vol. 1 and 2, Tokyo 1962.
146a. HEASMAN, M. A.: Accuracy of death certification. Proc. roy. Soc. Med. **55**, 733—736 (1962).
146b. —, and L. LIPWORTH: Accuracy of certification of cause of death. London H. M. Stationery Office 1966.
147. HECHTER, H., and N. O. BORHANI: Mortality and geographic distribution of arterio-sclerotic heart disease. Publ. Hlth Rep. **80**, 11—24 (1965).
148. HEYMAN, A.: (1) Natural history and clinical background of cerebrovascular disease. Publ. Hlth Monogr. **76**, 1—7 (1966).
149. —, W. G. YOUNG, JR., I. W. BROWN, JR., and K. S. GRIMSON: Long-term results of endarterectomy of the internal carotid artery for cerebral ischemia and infarction. Circulation **36**, 212—221 (1967).
150. —, M. D. NEFZGER, and E. H. ESTES: Serum cholesterol level in cerebral infarction. Arch. Neurol. (Chic.) **5**, 264—268 (1961).
151. —, H. A. SALTZMAN, and R. E. WHALEN: (2) The use of hyperbaric oxygenation in the treatment of cerebral ischemia and infarction. Circulation **33/34** (Suppl. II), II-20 to II-27 (1966).

152. HILL, A. B.: Statistical methods in clinical and preventive medicine. New York: Oxford Univ. Press 1962.

153. HILTNER, G., J. MÜLLER, G. DIPOL und H.-G. ZIELKE: Zur Frage der Ätiopathogenese zerebraler Gefäßprozesse bei Personen unter 50 Jahren. Z. ges. inn. Med. **19**, 318—323 (1964).

154. HOLMAN, R. L., and J. MOOSSY: The natural history of aortic, coronary and cerebral atherosclerosis (a preliminary report). In: FIELDS, W. S.: Pathogenesis and treatment of cerebrovascular disease, pp. 39—54. Springfield, Ill.: Charles C Thomas 1961.

155. House committee print no. 69: Historical statistics of the veteran population, 1865—1960 — A compendium of facts about veterans. Washington, D. C.: U.S. Govt. Printing Office 1961.

156. HOWARD, F. A., R. B. HICKLER, S. LOCKE, T. NEWCOMB, and H. R. TYLER: Survival following stroke. J. Amer. med. Ass. **183**, 921—925 (1963).

157. HOWARD, J.: Race differences in hypertension mortality trends. Differential drug exposure as a theory. Milbank mem. F. Quart. **43**, 202—218 (1965).

158. HOWELL, D. A., W. F. T. TATLOW, and S. FELDMAN: Observations on anticoagulant therapy in thromboembolic disease of the brain. Canad. med. Ass. J. **90**, 611—614 (1964).

159. HUSNI, E. A., H. S. BELL, and J. STORER: Mechanical occlusion of the vertebral artery. A new clinical concept. J. Amer. med. Ass. **196**, 475—478 (1966).

160. ILLIS, L., R. S. KOCEN, and W. I. McDONALD: Oral contraceptives and cerebral arterial occlusion. Brit. med. J. **1965 II**, 1164—1166.

161. JABLON, S., D. M. ANGEVINE, Y. S. MATSUMOTO, and M. ISHIDA: On the significance of cause of death as recorded on death certificates in Hiroshima and Nagasaki, Japan. Nat. Cancer Inst. Monogr. **19**, 445—465 (1966).

162. JAMES, G., R. E. PATTON, and A. S. HESLIN: Accuracy of cause-of-death statements on death certificates. Publ. Hlth Rep. **70**, 39—51 (1955).

163. JELLINEK, E. H., M. PAINTER, J. PRINEAS, and R. R. RUSSELL: Hypertensive encephalopathy with cortical disorders of vision. Quart. J. Med. **33**, 239—256 (1964).

163a. JENNETT, W. B., and J. N. CROSS: Influence of pregnancy and oral contraception on the incidence of strokes in women of childbearing age. Lancet **1967 I**, 1019—1023.

164. JOHNSON, K. G., K. YANO, and H. KATO: Cerebral vascular disease in Hiroshima, Japan. J. chron. Dis. **20**, 545—559 (1967).

165. JÖRGENSEN, L., and A. TORVIK: Ischaemic cerebrovascular diseases in an autopsy series. Part 1. Prevalence, location and predisposing factors in verified thrombo-embolic occlusions, and their significance in the pathogenesis of cerebral infarction. J. neurol. Sci. **3**, 490—509 (1966).

166. JUSTIN-BESANÇON, L., J. CHRÉTIEN et PH. DELAVIERRE: Causes de mortalité. Comparaison avec les statistiques officielles. Sem. Hôp. Paris **40**, 546—551 (1964).

167. —, PH. DELAVIERRE et J. CHRÉTIEN: Recherche des causes de mortalité à l'aide de 1000 confrontations anatomocliniques. Bull. Soc. Méd. Hôp. Paris **114**, 815—824 (1963).

168. KAHN, H. A.: The Dorn study of smoking and mortality among U.S. veterans: report on eight and one-half years of observation. Nat. Cancer Inst. Monogr. **19**, 1—125 (1966).

169. KANNEL, W. B.: An epidemiologic study of cerebrovascular disease. In: SIEKERT, R. G., and J. P. WHISNANT: Transactions of the fifth Princeton Conference, pp. 53—66. New York: Grune and Stratton 1966.

170. —, T. R. DAWBER, M. E. COHEN, and P. M. McNAMARA: Vascular disease of the brain — epidemiologic aspects: the Framingham study. Amer. J. publ. Hlth **55**, 1355—1366 (1965).

171. —, —, A. KAGAN, N. REVOTSKIE, and J. STOKES III.: Factors of risk in the development of coronary heart disease — six-year follow-up experience. The Framingham study, Ann. intern. Med. **55**, 33—50 (1961).

172. KATSUKI, S.: (1) Current concepts of the frequency of cerebral hemorrhage and cerebral infarction in Japan. In: SIEKERT, R. G., and J. P. WHISNANT: Transactions of the fifth Princeton Conference, pp. 99—111. New York: Grune and Stratton 1966.

173. KATSUKI S., and Y. HIROTA: (2) Recent trends in incidence of cerebral hemorrhage and infarction in Japan. A report based on death rate, autopsy case and prospective study on cerebro- vascular disease. Jap. Heart J. 7, 26—34 (1966).

174. — —, T. AKAZOME, S. TAKAYA, T. OMAE, and S. TAKANO: (1) Epidemiological studies on cerebrovascular diseases in Hisayama, Kyushu Island, Japan. Part I. With particular reference to cardiovascular status. Jap. Heart J. 5, 12—36 (1964).

175. —, T. OMAE, and Y. HIROTA: (2) Epidemiological and clinicopathological studies on cerebrovascular disease. Kyushu J. med. Sci. 15, 127—149 (1964).

176. —, H. UZAWA, S. FUJIMI, K. SHIRATSUCHI, and Y. ITO: (3) Studies on blood lipids in cases with cerebrovascular diseases. A preliminary report. Jap. Heart J. 5, 101—107 (1964).

177. KATZ, S., A. B. FORD, A. B. CHINN, and V. A. NEWILL: (Prognosis after strokes) Part II. Long-term course of 159 patients. Medicine (Baltimore) 45, 236—246 (1966).

178. KINSEY, D., H. S. SISE, and G. P. WHITELAW: Changes in mortality rates of treated hypertensive patients in a decade. Geriatrics 16, 397—415 (1961).

179. KNOWLER, L. A.: Some statistical aspects of a cooperative study. J. Neurosurg. 24, 789—791 (1966).

180. KNOX, G. S.: How often are we wrong ? or the epidemiology of doctor error. J. Okla. med. Ass. 57, 494—500 (1964).

181. KOHN, R. R.: Human aging and disease. J. chron. Dis. 16, 5—21 (1963).

182. KOJIMA, S., and R. KONISHI: Epidemiological studies on regional difference in apoplexy death rate in Akita prefecture. Tohoku J. exp. Med. 84, 166—198 (1964).

183. KRUEGER, D. E.: (1) New numerators for old denominators — multiple causes of death. Nat. Cancer Inst. Monogr. 19, 431—443 (1966).

184. — (2) Hypertensive and chronic respiratory disease mortality: confirmation of trends by multiple cause of death data. Publ. Hlth Rep. 81, 197—198 (1966).

185. —, J. L. WILLIAMS, and R. S. PAFFENBARGER JR.: Trends in death rates from cerebrovascular disease in Memphis, Tennessee, 1920—1960. J. chron. Dis. 20, 129—137 (1967).

186. Kungl. Medicinalstyrelsen: Allmän Hälso-och Sjukvård år 1928—1933. Stockholm: P. A. Norstedt and Söner 1930—1935.

187. KURLAND, L. T.: Descriptive epidemiology of selected neurologic and myopathic disorders with particular reference to a survey in Rochester, Minnesota. J. chron. Dis. 8, 378—418 (1958).

188. —, N. W. CHOI, and G. P. SAYRE: Current status of the epidemiology of cerebrovascular diseases. In: FIELDS, W. S., and W. A. SPENCER (Ed.): Stroke rehabilitation: Basic concepts and research trends, pp. 3—22 (1967).

189. KURZTKE, J. F.: Medical facilities and the prevalence of multiple sclerosis. Acta neurol. scand. 41, 561—579 (1965).

190. — (1) An evaluation of the geographic distribution of multiple sclerosis. Acta neurol. scand. 42, suppl. 19, 91—117 (1966).

191. — (2) An epidemiologic approach to multiple sclerosis. Arch. Neurol. (Chic.) 14, 213—222 (1966).

192. — (3) The distribution of multiple sclerosis and other diseases. Acta neurol. scand. 42, 221—243 (1966).

193. — (4) On statistical testing of prevalence studies. J. chron. Dis. 19, 909—922 (1966).

194. — Further considerations on the geographic distribution of multiple sclerosis. Acta neurol. scand. 43, 283—298 (1967).

195. LADD, A. C.: Cerebrovascular disease in an employed population. J. chron. Dis. 15, 985—990 (1962).

196.* LANDAU, W. M., F. H. McDOWELL, G. L. ODOM, and R. P. SCHMIDT (Ed.): Proceedings of International Conference on Vascular Disease of the Brain, Neurology 11, part 2, Minneapolis: Lancet Publications 1961.

197. LARRSON, T.: Mortality from cerebrovascular disease. In: ENGEL, A., and T. LARRSON: Thule International Symposia. Stroke, pp. 15—40 (1967).

198. LAURSSEN, J.: Personal communication, Danmarks Statistiske Departement, May 1963.

199. LEISHMAN, A. W. D.: Merits of reducing high blood-pressure. Lancet 1963 I, 1284—1288.

200. LILIENFELD, A. M.: Workshop on the epidemiology of cerebrovascular disease. Publ. Hlth Monogr. **76**, 65—69 (1966).
201. LINDGREN, S. O.: Course and prognosis in spontaneous occlusions of cerebral arteries. Acta psychiat. neurol. Scand. **33**, 343—358 (1958).
202. LINELL, F., and J. SÖDERSTRÖM: Synpunkter på värdet av dödsorsaks- och sjukdomsstatistik. Svenska Läk-Tidn. **60**, 2895—2901 (1963).
203. LOCKSLEY, H. B.: (1) Report on the cooperative study of intracranial aneurysms and subarachnoid hemorrhage. Section V, Part I. Natural history of subarachnoid hemorrhage, intracranial aneurysms, and arteriovenous malformations based on 6368 cases in the cooperative study. J. Neurosurg. **25**, 219—239 (1966).
204. — (2) Report on the cooperative study of intracranial aneurysms and subarachnoid hemorrhage. Section V, Part II. J. Neurosurg. **25**, 321—368 (1966).
205. —, A. L. SAHS, and L. KNOWLER: (3) Report on the cooperative study of intracranial aneurysms and subarachnoid hemorrhage. Section II. General survey of cases in the central registry and characteristics of the sample population. J. Neurosurg. **24**, 922—932 (1966).
206. — —, and R. SANDLER: (4) Report on the cooperative study of intracranial aneurysms and subarachnoid hemorrhage. Section III. Subarachnoid hemorrhage unrelated to intracranial aneurysm and A-V malformation. A study of associated diseases and prognosis. J. Neurosurg. **24**, 1034—1056 (1966).
207. LOGAN, W. P. D., and A. A. CUSHION: Studies on medical and population subjects no. 14. Morbidity statistics from general practice, Vol. I (General). London: H. M. Stationery Office 1958.
208. LOUIS, S., and F. MCDOWELL: Stroke in young adults. Ann. intern. Med. **66**, 932—938 (1967).
209. LYONS, C.: Progress report of the joint study of extracranial arterial occlusion. In: MILLIKAN, C. H., R. G. SIEKERT, and J. P. WHISNANT: Cerebral vascular diseases, pp. 221—239. New York: Grune and Stratton 1965.
210. MAGEE, C. G.: Spontaneous subarachnoid hemorrhage. A review of 150 cases. Lancet **1943 II**, 497—500.
211. MAINLAND, D.: Elementary medical statistics. The principles of quantitative medicine. Philadelphia: W. B. Saunders Co. 1952.
212. — Elementary medical statistics, 2nd ed. Philadelphia: W. B. Saunders Co. 1963.
213. MARGOLIS, G.: The vascular changes and pathogenesis of hypertensive intracerebral hemorrhage. Ass. Res. nerv. ment. Dis. Proc. **41**, 73—91 (1966).
214. —, G. L. ODOM, and B. WOODHALL: Further experiences with small vascular malformations as a cause of massive intracerebral bleeding. J. Neuropath. exp. Neurol. **20**, 161—167 (1961).
215. MARMORSTON, J.: Effect of estrogen treatment in cerebrovascular disease. In: MILLIKAN, C. H., R. G. SIEKERT, and J. P. WHISNANT: Cerebral vascular diseases, pp. 214—221. New York: Grune and Stratton 1965.
216. MARSHALL, J.: Hypertension and cerebrovascular disease. Proc. roy. Soc. Med. **56**, 486—487 (1963).
217. — (1) The natural history of transient ischaemic cerebro-vascular attacks. Quart. J. Med. **33**, 309—324 (1964).
218. — (2) A trial of long-term hypotensive therapy in cerebrovascular disease. Lancet **1964 I**, 10—12.
219. — The prevention of strokes. Amer Heart J. **71**, 1—4 (1966).
220. —, and A. C. KAESER: Survival after non-haemorrhagic cerebrovascular accidents, a prospective study. Brit. med. J. **1961 II**, 73—77.
221. —, and E. H. REYNOLDS: Withdrawal of anticoagulants from patients with transient ischaemic cerebrovascular attacks. Lancet **1965 I**, 5—6.
222. —, and D. A. SHAW: The natural history of cerebrovascular disease. Brit. med. J. **1959 I**, 1614—1617.
223. MARTIN, M. J., G. P. SAYRE, and J. P. WHISNANT: Incidence of occlusive vascular disease in the extracranial arteries contributing to the cerebral circulation. Trans. Amer. neurol. Ass. **85**, 103—105 (1960).

224. Mathai, K. V., and J. Chandy: Incidence of subarachnoid haemorrhage. Neurology India (Bombay) 13, 40—41 (1965).

225.* May, J. M.: The ecology of human disease. M D Publications, New York 1958.

226.* — (Ed.): Studies in disease ecology. New York: Hafner Publ. Co. 1961.

227. McCormick, W. F.: The pathology of vascular ("arteriovenous") malformations. J. Neurosurg. 24, 807—816 (1966).

228. McDevitt, E., S. A. Carter, B. W. Gatje, W. T. Foley, and I. S. Wright: Use of anticoagulants in treatment of cerebral vascular disease. Ten-year experience in treatment of thromboembolism. J. Amer. med. Ass. 166, 592—597 (1958).

229. McDonough, J. R.: Field epidemiology applied to chronic diseases. Georgetown med. Bull. 19, 128—136, 179—197 (1966).

230. McDowell, F., and E. McDevitt: Treatment of the completed stroke with long-term anticoagulant: six and one-half years experience. In: Millikan, C. H., R. G. Siekert, and J. P. Whisnant: Cerebral vascular diseases, pp. 185—199. New York: Grune and Stratton 1965.

231. —, J. Potes, and S. Groch: The natural history of internal carotid and vertebral-basilar artery occlusion. Neurology (Minneap.) 11, (part 2) 153—157 (1961).

232. McGandy, R. B., D. M. Hegsted, and F. J. Stare: Dietary fats, carbohydrates and atherosclerotic vascular disease. New Engl. J. Med. 277, 186—192, 242—247 (1967).

233. McKissock, W., K. Paine, and L. Walsh: Further observations on subarachnoid haemorrhage. J. Neurol. Neurosurg. Psychiat. 21, 239—248 (1958).

234. —, A. Richardson, and L. Walsh: "Posterior-communicating" aneurysms. A controlled trial of conservative and surgical treatment of ruptured aneurysms of the internal carotid artery at or near the point of origin of the posterior communicating artery. Lancet 1960 I, 1203—1206.

235. — — — Middle-cerebral aneurysms. Further results in the controlled trial of conservative and surgical treatment of ruptured intracranial aneurysms. Lancet 1962 II, 417—421.

236. — — — Anterior communicating aneurysms. A trial of conservative and surgical treatment. Lancet 1965 I, 873—876.

237. — — —, and E. Owen: Multiple intracranial aneurysms. Lancet 1964 I, 623—626.

238. McMurtry, J. G. III, J. L. Pool, and H. R. Nova: The use of Rheomacrodex in the surgery of intracranial aneurysms. J. Neurosurg. 26, 218—222 (1967).

239. Merrett, J. D., and G. F. Adams: Comparison of mortality rates in elderly hypertensive and normotensive hemiplegic patients. Brit. med. J. 1966 II, 802—805.

240. Meyer, J. S.: The neurological examination, diagnosis, and prevention of strokes. In: DeForest, R. E.: Proceedings of the National Stroke Congress, pp. 65—70. Springfield, Ill.: Charles C Thomas 1966.

241. —, J. Gilroy, M. E. Barnhart, and J. F. Johnson: Therapeutic thrombolysis in cerebral thromboembolism: randomized evaluation of intravenous streptokinase. In: Millikan, C. H., R. G. Siekert, and J. P. Whisnant: Cerebral vascular diseases, pp. 200—213. New York: Grune and Stratton 1965.

242. —, A. G. Waltz, J. W. Hess, and B. Zak: Serum lipid and cholesterol levels in cerebrovascular disease. Arch. Neurol. (Chic.) 1, 303—311 (1959).

243. Miall, W. E., and H. G. Lovell: Relation between change of blood pressure and age. Brit. med. J. 1967 II, 660—664.

244. Millikan, C. H.: Anticoagulant therapy in cerebrovascular disease. In: Millikan, C. H., R. G. Siekert, and J. P. Whisnant: Cerebral vascular diseases, pp. 181—184. New York: Grune and Stratton 1961.

245. — (1) Diagnosis of the stroke-prone patient. In: DeForest, R. E.: Proceedings of the National Stroke Congress, pp. 44—49. Springfield, Ill.: Charles C Thomas 1966.

246.* — (2) Cerebrovascular disease. Science 152, 803—807 (1966).

247.* — (Ed.): (3) Cerebrovascular disease. Ass. Res. nerv. ment. Dis. Proc. 41 (1966).

248. —, and F. P. Moersch: Factors that influence prognosis in acute focal cerebrovascular lesions. Arch. Neurol. Psychiat. (Chic.) 70, 558—562 (1953).

249.* —, R. G. Siekert, and J. P. Whisnant: Cerebral vascular diseases. Transactions of the third Conference, January 4—6, 1961. New York: Grune and Stratton 1961.

250.* MILLIKAN C. H., R. G. SIEKERT, and J. P. WHISNANT: Cerebral vascular diseases. Transactions of the fourth Conference, January 8—10, 1964. New York: Grune and Stratton 1965.

251. Ministry of Health and Welfare, Japanese Government: A Brief Report on Public Health Administration in Japan, 1962. Tokyo 1962.

252. MOHLER, E. R. JR., and E. D. FREIS: Five-year survival of patients with malignant hypertension treated with antihypertensive agents. Amer. Heart J. **60**, 329—335 (1960).

253. MOOSSY, J.: Development of cerebral atherosclerosis in various age groups. Neurology (Minneap.) **9**, 569—574 (1959).

254. — Cerebral infarcts and complicated lesions of intracranial and extracranial atherosclerosis. In: MILLIKAN, C. H., R. G. SIEKERT, and J. P. WHISNANT: Cerebral vascular diseases, pp. 162—167. New York: Grune and Stratton 1965.

255. — (1) Morphology, sites and epidemiology of cerebral atherosclerosis. Ass. res. nerv. ment. Dis. Proc. **41**, 1—22 (1966).

256. — (2) Cerebral infarction and intracranial arterial thrombosis. Necropsy studies and clinical implications. Arch. Neurol. (Chic.) **14**, 119—123 (1966).

257. — (3) Cerebral infarcts and the lesions of intracranial and extracranial atherosclerosis. Arch. Neurol. (Chic.) **14**, 124—128 (1966).

258. MORIYAMA, I. M., W. S. BAUM, W. M. HAENSZEL, and B. F. MATTISON: Inquiry into diagnostic evidence supporting medical certifications of death. Amer. J. publ. Hlth. **48**, 1376—1387 (1958).

259. —, T. R. DAWBER, and W. B. KANNEL: Evaluation of diagnostic information supporting medical certification of deaths from cardiovascular disease. Nat. Cancer Inst. Monogr. **19**, 405—409 (1966).

260. MORRIS, J. N., M. D. CRAWFORD, and J. A. HEADY: Hardness of local water-supplies and mortality from cardiovascular disease. Lancet **1961 I**, 860—862; **1962 II**, 506—507.

261. MOUREN, P., A. TATOSSIAN, R. TRUPHEME, P. GUIN, and M. ROBION: Etude statistique du pronostic vital à court terme des accidents vasculaires cérébraux communs. Marseille-méd. **102**, 699—713 (1965).

262. MULCAHY, R.: The influence of water hardness and rainfall on the incidence of cardiovascular and cerebrovascular mortality in Ireland. J. Irish med. Ass. **55**, 17—18 (1964).

263. MUNCK, W.: Autopsy finding and clinical diagnosis. A comparative study of 1000 cases. Acta med. scand. **142**, suppl. 266, 775—781 (1952).

264. MURPHEY, F., and D. A. MacCUBBIN: Carotid endarterectomy. A long-term follow-up study. J. Neurosurg. **23**, 156—168 (1965).

265. NAIK, B. K., P. S. RAO, and R. SABOO: Incidence of ischaemic heart disease and cerebrovascular disease in Hyderabad. Indian Heart J. **18**, 37—44 (1966).

266.* NEEL, J. V., M. W. SHAW, and W. J. SCHULL: Genetics and the Epidemiology of Chronic Diseases, U.S.P.H.S. Division of Chronic Diseases, P.H.S. Publication No. 1163. Washington, D.C.: U.S. Govt. Printing Office 1965.

267. NEFZGER, M. D., A. HEYMAN, J. LeBAUER, S. FRIEDBERG, and J. LEWIS: Serum cholesterol levels in myocardial and cerebral infarction caused by atherosclerosis. J. Chron. Dis. **20**, 593—602 (1967).

268. NEWELL, D. J.: Errors in the interpretation of errors in epidemiology. Amer. J. publ. Hlth **52**, 1925—1928 (1962).

269. NICHAMAN, M. Z., E. BOYLE JR., T. P. LESESNE, and H. I. SAUER: Cardiovascular disease mortality by race. Based on a statistical study in Charleston, South Carolina. Geriatrics **17**, 724—737 (1962).

270. NISHIOKA, H.: Report on the cooperative study of intracranial aneurysms and subarachnoid hemorrhage. Section VII, Part I. Evaluation of the conservative management of ruptured intracranial aneurysms. J. Neurosurg. **25**, 574—592 (1966).

271. O'BRIEN, M. D., N. VEALL, R. J. LUCK, and W. T. IRVINE: Cerebral-cortex perfusion-rates in extracranial cerebrovascular disease and the effects of operation. Lancet **1967 II**, 392—395.

272. OJEMANN, R. G.: The surgical treatment of cerebrovascular disease. New Engl. J. Med. **274**, 440—448 (1966).

273. O'Leary, J.: Cerebrovascular diseases. Epidemiology. Nat. Conf. Cardiovasc. Dis. 2, 424—425 (1964).
274. Olson, F. E., F. D. Norris, L. M. Hammes, and B. A. Shipley: A study of multiple causes of death in California. J. chron. Dis. 15, 157—170 (1962).
275. Ostfeld, A. M.: Are strokes preventable? Med. Clin. N. Amer. 51, 105—111 (1967).
276. Otterland, A., and E. Pihl: Klinisk patologisk-anatomisk och officiell dödsorsaks-diagnostik med utgängspunkt från 327 obductionsfall. Svenska Läk-Tidn. 61, 68—86 (1964).
277. Paffenbarger, R. S., R. N. Milling, N. D. Poe, and D. E. Krueger: (1) Trends in death rates from hypertensive disease in Memphis, Tennessee, 1920—1960. J. chron. Dis. 19, 847—856 (1966).
278. —, J. Notkin, D. E. Krueger, P. A. Wolf, M. C.Thorne, E. J. LeBauer, and J. L. Williams: (2) Chronic disease in former college students. II. Methods of study and observations on mortality from coronary heart disease. Amer. J. publ. Hlth 56, 962—971 (1966).
279. —, and J. L. Williams: (1) Chronic disease in former college students. V. Early precursors of fatal stroke. J. chron. Dis. 57, 1290—1299 (1967).
280. —, and A. L. Wing: (2) Characteristics in youth predisposing to fatal stroke in later years. Lancet 1967 I, 753—754.
281. —, P. A. Wolf, J. Notkin, and M. C. Thorne: (3) Chronic disease in former college students. I. Early precursors of fatal coronary heart disease. Amer. J. Epidem. 83, 314—328 (1966).
282. Pakarinen, S.: Incidence, aetiology, and prognosis of primary subarachnoid haemorrhage. A study based on 589 cases diagnosed in a defined urban population during a defined period. Acta neurol. scand. 43, suppl. 29, 1—128 (1967).
283. Parrish, H. M., G. H. Payne, W. C. Allen, J. C. Goldner, and H. I. Sauer: Mid-Missouri stroke survey; a preliminary report. Missouri Med. 1966, 816—821.
284.* Paul, J. R.: Clinical epidemiology (Revised Edition). Chicago, Ill.: University of Chicago Press 1966.
285. Paul, O., and A. M. Ostfeld: Epidemiology of hypertension. Progr. cardiovasc. Dis. 8, 106—116 (1965).
286. Pearce, J. M. S., S. S. Gubbay, and J. N. Walton: Long-term anticoagulant therapy in transient cerebral ischaemic attacks. Lancet 1965 I, 6—9.
287. Pell, S., and C. A. D'Alonzo: Acute myocardial infarction in a large industrial population. Report of a 6-year study of 1,356 cases. J. Amer. med. Ass. 185, 831—838 (1963).
288. — — Some aspects of hypertension in diabetes mellitus. J. Amer. med. Ass. 202, 10—16 (1967).
289. Pemberton, J. (Ed.): Epidemiology. Reports on research and teaching 1962. London: Oxford University Press 1963.
290. Pennybacker, J.: The surgical aspects of strokes. Proc. roy. Soc. Med. 56, 487—488 (1963).
291. Perret, G., and H. Nishioka: (1) Report on the cooperative study of intracranial aneurysms and subarachnoid hemorrhage. Section IV. Cerebral angiography. An analysis of the diagnostic value and complications of carotid and vertebral angiography in 5,484 patients. J. Neurosurg. 25, 98—114 (1966).
292. — — (2) Report on the cooperative study of intracranial aneurysms and subarachnoid hemorrhage. Section VI. Arteriovenous malformations. An analysis of 545 cases of cranio-cerebral arteriovenous malformations and fistulae reported to the cooperative study. J. Neurosurg. 25, 467—490 (1966).
293. Peters, C. C., and W. R. Van Voorhis: Statistical procedures and their mathematical bases. New York: McGraw-Hill Book Co. 1940.
294. Pincock, J. G.: The natural history of cerebral thrombosis. Ann. intern. Med. 46, 925—930 (1957).
295. Pohlen, K., and H. Emerson: Errors in clinical statements of causes of death. Amer. J. publ. Hlth 32, 251—260 (1942).
296. — — Errors in clinical statements of causes of death. Second report. Amer. J. publ. Hlth 33, 505—516 (1943).

297. POOL, J. L., and R. P. COLTON: Anterior communicating aneurysms. A rebuttal. J. Amer. med. Ass. **195**, 115—116 (1966).
298.* The President's Commission on Heart Disease, Cancer and Stroke. Report to the President. A National Program to Conquer Heart Disease, Cancer, and Stroke, Vol. I, Vol. II. Washington, D.C.: U.S. Govt. Printing Office 1964/1965.
299.* Public Health Service: Cerebrovascular Disease Epidemiology. A Workshop, Publ. Health Monogr. No. 76 (PHS Publication No. 1441). Washington, D.C.: U.S. Govt. Printing Office 1966.
300. RAMAMURTHI, B.: Are subarachnoid haemorrhages uncommon in India. Neurol. India **13**, 42—43 (1965).
301. REID, D. D., and G. A. ROSE: Assessing the comparability of mortality statistics. Brit. med. J. **1964 II**, 1437—1439.
302. REIVICH, M., H. E. HOLLING, B. ROBERTS, and J. F. TOOLE: Reversal of blood flow through the vertebral artery and its effect on cerebral circulation. New Engl. J. Med. **265**, 878—885 (1961).
303. Research Committee of the Council of the College of General Practitioners: Studies on Medical and Population Subjects. No. 14. Morbidity Statistics from General Practice III (Disease in General Practice). London: H. M. Stationery Office 1962.
304. REUTER, J. P.: Disponierende und auslösende Faktoren in der Pathogenese und Ätiologie des Schlaganfalls. Dtsch. med. J. **15**, 77—98 (1964).
305. RICHARDSON, A. E., J. A. JANE, and P. M. PAYNE: The prediction of morbidity and mortality in anterior communicating aneurysms treated by proximal anterior cerebral ligation. J. Neurosurg. **25**, 280—283 (1966).
306. ROB, C. G., and J. A. DeWEESE: Surgical treatment of transient strokes. Postgrad. Med. **42**, 19—22 (1967).
307. ROBINSON, R. W., W. D. COHEN, N. HIGANO, R. MEYER, G. H. LUKOWSKY, R. B. Mc LAUGHLIN, and H. H. MACGILPIN: Life-table analysis of survival after cerebral thrombosis — ten-year experience. J. Amer. med. Ass. **169**, 1149—1152 (1959).
308. —, N. HIGANO, and W. D. COHEN: Comparison of serum lipid levels in patients with cerebral thrombosis and in normal subjects. Ann. intern. Med. **59**, 180—185 (1963).
309. ROSE, G.: (1) Cardiovascular mortality among American Negroes. Arch. environm. Hlth **5**, 412—414 (1962).
310. — (2) The distribution of mortality from hypertension within the United States. J. chron. Dis. **15**, 1017—1024 (1962).
311. ROSS, G. S.: Transient ischemic attacks. Stroke **1**, 1—4 (1966).
312. — Personal communication, Syracuse, New York, August 11. (1967).
313. SAHS, A. L.: (1) Observations on the pathology of saccular aneurysms. J. Neurosurg. **24**, 792—806 (1966).
314. — (2) Report on the cooperative study of intracranial aneurysms and subarachnoid hemorrhage. Section VII, Part 2. Hypotension and hypothermia in the treatment of intracranial aneurysms. J. Neurosurg. **25**, 593—600 (1966).
315. —, G. PERRET, H. B. LOCKSLEY, H. NISHIOKA, and F. M. SKULTETY: (3) Report on the cooperative study of intracranial aneurysms and subarachnoid hemorrhage. I. Preliminary remarks on subarachnoid hemorrhage. J. Neurosurg. **24**, 782—788 (1966).
316. SARNER, M., and M. D. CRAWFORD: Ruptured intracranial aneurysm. Clinical series. Lancet **1965 II**, 1251—1254.
317. —, and F. C. ROSE: Clinical presentation of ruptured intracranial aneurysm. J. Neurol. Neurosurg. Psychiat. **30**, 67—70 (1967).
318. SCHROEDER, H. A.: Degenerative cardiovascular disease in the Orient: hypertension. J. chron. Dis. **8**, 312—333 (1958).
319. — Relations between hardness of water and death rates from certain chronic and degenerative diseases in the United States. J. chron. Dis. **12**, 586—591 (1960).
320. — Municipal drinking water and cardiovascular death rates. J. Amer. med. Ass. **195**, 81—85 (1966).
321. SCOTCH, N. A., and H. J. GEIGER: The epidemiology of essential hypertension. A review with special attention to psychologic and sociocultural factors. II: Psychologic and sociocultural factors in etiology. J. chron. Dis. **16**, 1183—1213 (1963).

322. SHAFEY, S., and P. SCHEINBERG: Neurological syndromes occuring in patients receiving synthetic steroids (oral contraceptives). Neurology (Minneap.) **16**, 205—211 (1966).
323. SHENKIN, H. A., H. HAFT, and F. M. SOMACH: Prognostic significance of arteriography in nonhemorrhagic strokes. J. Amer. med. Ass. **194**, 612—616 (1965).
324. SIEGEL, S.: Nonparametric statistics for the behavioral sciences. New York: McGraw-Hill Book Co. 1956.
325.* SIEKERT, R. G., and J. P. WHISNANT (Ed.): Cerebral vascular diseases. Transactions of the Fifth Conference January 5—7, 1966. New York: Grune and Stratton 1966. (Note: this work is also cited as MILLIKAN, SIEKERT, and WHISNANT; Dr. MILLIKAN is the chairman of this series of works since the third conference.)
326. — —, and C. H. MILLIKAN: Surgical and anticoagulant therapy of occlusive cerebrovascular disease. Ann. intern. Med. **58**, 637—641 (1963).
327. SIRKEN, M. G.: The potential impact [of the decennial undercount] on vital statistics, Washington Statistical Society meeting, October 25, Washington, D.C. (1967).
328. SJÖSTRÖM, Å.: Hospitalized cases of stroke in a Swedish hospital region. In: ENGEL, A., and T. LARRSON, Thule International Symposia. Stroke, pp. 41—50 (1967).
329. SKYRING, A., B. MODAN, A. CROCETTI, and C. HAMMERSTROM: Some epidemiological and familial aspects of coronary heart disease: report of a pilot study. J. chron. Dis. **16**, 1267—1279 (1963).
330. SMIRK, H., and J. V. HODGE: Causes of death in treated hypertensive patients based on 82 deaths during 1959—1961 among an average hypertensive population at risk of 518 persons. Brit. med. J. **1963 II**, 1221—1225.
331. SNEDECOR, G. W.: Statistical methods applied to experiments in agriculture and biology. 5. Ed. Ames, Iowa: Iowa State University Press 1956.
332. SNOW, J.: Snow on cholera. Being a reprint of two papers (facsimile of the 1936 edition). New York: Hafner Publishing Co. 1965.
333. SODELAND, P.: Personal communication. Division of hygiene and epidemiology. Health Services of Norway, Oslo, July 7. 1964.
334. SOX, E. D., and M. HOLATA: Underlying causes of death, cardiovascular disease. San Francisco experience in the Pan American Health Organization international mortality study, presented at the Epidemiology and Statistics Sections, 94th annual meeting A.P.H.A., October 31. 1966.
335. STAMLER, J.: Epidemiology of cerebrovascular diseases. In: DEFOREST, R. E., Proceedings of the National Stroke Congress, pp. 24—37. Springfield, Ill.: Charles C Thomas 1966.
336. STALLONES, R. A.: Epidemiology of cerebrovascular disease. A review. J. chron. Dis. **18**, 859—872 (1965).
337. — Prospective epidemiologic studies of cerebrovascular disease. Publ. Hlth Monogr. **76**, 51—55 (1966).
338. Statistisk Sentralbyrå: Folkemengdens Bevegelse 1946. Oslo: H. Aschehoug & Co. 1949.
339. — Statistisk Årbok for Norge 65. 67. Årgang 1946—1948. Oslo: H. Aschehoug & Co. 1948.
340. — Sunnhetstilstanden og Medisinalforholdene 1946, 1947, 1948, 94., 95., 96. Årgang. Oslo: H. Aschehoug & Co. 1949/1950.
341. Statistiska Centralbyrån: Dödsorsaker År 1933, 1960. Stockholm: P. A. Norstedt & Söner 1936/1960.
342. — Dödsorsaksmönstret i Sverige under 1950-Talet, Stockholm (1966).
343. — Dödligheten i Länen 1959—1962. Stockholm: Svenska Reproduktions AB, 1964.
344. — Statistisk Årsbok för Sverige. Tjugoförsta Årgangen 1934. Stockholm: P. A. Norsted & Söner, 1934.
345. — Statistisk Årsbok för Sverige. Tjugoandra Årgangen 1935. Stockholm: P. A. Norstedt & Söner, 1935.
346. — Statistisk Årsbok för Sverige. Årgangen 47, 1960. Stockholm: P. A. Norstedt & Söner, 1960.
347. Det Statistiske Departement: Danmarks Statistik: Statistik Årbog 1921, 1938, 1948 (53 Aargang), 1962 (vol. 67). Copenhagen (1921, 1938, 1948, 1963).

348. Sugita, K., E. Kimura, T. Tsuda, T. Sakakibara, and R. Ushiku: Lost years of life for index of mortality from cerebral apoplexy in the City of Yokohama. Yokohama med. Bull. 14, 115—122 (1963).

349. Sundhedsstyrelsen: Dødsårsagerne i Kongeriget Danmark 1950 (H. Hagerup), 1956 (Kgl. Hofbogtrykkeri), 1957—1960 (Statens Trykningskontor), Kobenhavn (1951, 1958 to 1961).

350. — Danmark: Medicinalberetning for Kongeriget Danmark i Året 1940, 1950. København: H. Hagerup, 1942, 1952.

351. Surawicz, B.: Electrocardiographic pattern of cerebrovascular accident. J. Amer. med. Ass. 197, 913—914 (1966).

352. Svein, H. J., and J. A. McRae: Arteriovenous anomalies of the brain. Fate of patients not having definitive surgery. J. Neurosurg. 23, 23—28 (1965).

353. —, I. Olive, and P. Angulo-Rivero: The fate of patients who have cerebral arteriovenous anomalies without definitive surgical treatments. J. Neurosurg. 13, 381—387 (1956).

354. Swartout, H. O., and R. G. Webster: To what degree are mortality statistics dependable? Amer. J. publ. Hlth 30, 811—815 (1940).

355. Takahashi, E. et. al.: Epidemiological studies on hypertension and cerebral hemorrhage in North-east Japan. Tohoku J. exp. Med. 74, 188—210 (1961).

356. —, N. Sasaki, J. Takeda, and H. Ito: The geographic distribution of cerebral hemorrhage and hypertension in Japan. Hum. Biol. 29, 139—166 (1957).

357. Tate, M. W., and R. C. Clelland: Nonparametric and shortcut statistics in the social, biological, and medical sciences. Danville, Ill.: Interstate Printers and Publishers, 1957.

358. Taylor, I., and J. Knowelden: Principles of epidemiology, 2. Ed. Boston: Little, Brown, & Co., 1964.

359. Tennent, E. C., and J. W. Harman: A study of factors affecting the prognosis of cerebral vascular accident. Amer. J. med. Sci. 218, 361—368 (1949).

360. Thompson, J. E., D. J. Austin, and R. D. Patman: Endarterectomy of the totally occluded carotid artery for stroke. Results in 100 operations. Arch. Surg. 95, 791—801 (1967).

361. —, M. M. Kartchner, D. J. Austin, C. G. Wheeler, and R. D. Patman: Clinical considerations in the surgical management of strokes. Circulation 33—34: suppl. I: I-162—I-172 (1966).

362. Thorner, R. M.: A cohort study of the blood pressure of 444 healthy white males. J. chron. Dis. 15, 117—130 (1962).

363. Tindall, G. T., J. A. Goree, J. F. Lee, and G. L. Odom: Effect of common carotid ligation on size of internal carotid aneurysms and distal intracarotid and retinal artery pressures. J. Neurosurg. 25, 503—511 (1966).

364.* Toole, J. F., and A. N. Patel: Cerebrovascular disorders: with sections on applied vascular anatomy and physiology of the brain and spinal cord. New York: Blakiston, 1967.

365. Trombold, J. C., R. C. Moellering, and A. Kagan: Epidemiological aspects of coronary heart disease and cerebrovascular disease: the Honolulu heart program. Hawaii med. J. 25, 231—234 (1966).

366. Trumpy, J. H.: Subarachnoid hemorrhage. Time sequence of recurrences and their prognosis. Acta neurol. scand. 43, 48—60 (1967).

367. Udall, J. A.: Anticoagulant therapy for progressing strokes. A guide for patient selection. Postgrad. Med. 42, 212—217 (1967).

368. Ueda, H. et. al.: Committee report. I. The epidemiologic survey of ischemic heart disease in Japan. II. The evaluation of anticoagulant therapy for myocardial infarction. Jap. Heart J. 5, 549—557 (1964).

369. Uihlein, A., R. L. Thomas, and J. Cleary: Aneurysms of the anterior communicating artery complex. Mayo Clin. Proc. 42, 73—87 (1967).

370. U.S. Bureau of the Census: Statistical abstract of the United States, 1961, 1964. Washington, D.C.: U.S. Govt. Printing Office, 1961, 1964.

371. — Historical statistics of the United States, 1957. Washington, D.C.: U.S. Govt. Printing Office, 1957.

372. U.S. Bureau of the Census: 1960 census of population. Alphabetical index of occupations and Industries (Revised Edition). Washington, D.C.: U.S. Govt. Printing Office, 1960.

373. — The statistical history of the United States from Colonial Times to the Present. Stamford, Conn.: Fairfield Publishers Inc., 1965.

374. Veterans Administration Cooperative Study of Atherosclerosis, Neurology Section: An evaluation of estrogenic substances in the treatment of cerebral vascular disease. Circulation **33—34**: (suppl. II) II-3—II-9 (1966).

375. VON HOFSTEN, E. Dödsorsaksstatistikens problem och möjligheter. Svenska. Lak.-Tidn. **61**, 24—35 (1964).

376. WAALER, E., and M. GRIMSTVEDT: The clinical diagnoses of the causes of death and their reliability. Acta path. microbiol. scand. **43**, 330—338 (1958).

377. WAKSBERG, J.: The dimensions of the decennial undercount, Washington Statistical Society meeting, October 25, Washington, D.C., 1967.

378. WALKER, A. R. P.: Mortality from coronary heart disease and from cerebral vascular disease in the different racial populations in South Africa. S. Afr. med. J. **37**, 1155 to 1159 (1963).

379. WALLACE, D. C. et. al.: Study of the natural history of cerebral vascular disease. Med. J. Austr. **1**, 90—95 (1967).

380. WALTON, J. N.: The late prognosis of subarachnoid haemorrhage. Brit. med. J. **1952 II**, 802—808.

381. WEIBEL, J., W. S. FIELDS, and R. J. CAMPOS: Aneurysms of the posterior cervicocranial circulation: clinical and angiographic considerations. J. Neurosurg. **26**, 223—234 (1967).

382. WELLS, C. E.: Cerebral embolism: the natural history, prognostic signs, and effects of anticoagulation. Arch. Neurol. Psychiat. (Chic.) **81**, 667—677 (1959).

383. —, and R. J. TIMBERGER: Cerebral thrombosis in patients under fifty years of age. Arch. Neurol. (Chic.) **4**, 268—271 (1961).

384. WHISNANT, J. P.: Cerebrovascular diseases: natural history. Publ. Hlth Monogr. **76**, 9—21 (1966).

385. —, R. G. SIEKERT, and C. H. MILLIKAN: Diagnosis and management of cerebral vascular disease: a review. J. Ark. med. Soc. **60**, 95—99 (1963).

386. WILLIAMS, D., and T. G. WILSON: The diagnosis of the major and minor syndromes of basilar insufficiency. Brain **85**, 741—774 (1962).

387. WINKELSTEIN, W.: Some retrospective studies of cerebrovascular disease. Publ. Hlth Monogr. **76**, 41—49 (1966).

388. WISOFF, H. S., and A. B. ROTHBALLER: Cerebral arterial thrombosis in children. Review of literature and addition of two cases in apparently healthy children. Arch. Neurol. (Chic.) **4**, 258—267 (1961).

389. WITTS, L. J.: Medical surveys and clinical trials. Some methods and applications of group research in medicine, 2. Ed. London: Oxford University Press, 1964.

390. WOLF, G.: Langfristige Beobachtungen bei Kranken mit Subarachnoidealblutungen (Vorläufige Mitteilung). Nervenarzt **34**, 73—76 (1963).

391. WOLF, G. A., JR., H. GOODELL, and H. G. WOLFF: Prognosis of subarachnoid hemorrhage and its relation to long term management. J. Amer. med. Ass. **129**, 715—718 (1945).

392. World Health Organization: Epidemiological and vital statistics reports. Vol. I—III. Geneva (1947—1950).

393. — International classification of diseases. Manual of the International Statistical Classification of Diseases, Injuries, and Causes of Death, Volume 1. Geneva (1957).

394.* WRIGHT, I. S., and E. H. LUCKEY: Cerebral vascular diseases. Transactions of the First Conference January 24—26, 1954. New York: Grune and Stratton, 1955.

395.* —, and C. H. MILLIKAN: Cerebral vascular diseases. Transactions of the Second Conference January 16—18, 1957. New York: Grune and Stratton, 1958.

396. WYLIE, C. M.: Recent trends in mortality from cerebrovascular accidents in the United States. J. chron. Dis. **14**, 213—220 (1961).

397. — (1) Cerebrovascular accident deaths in the United States and in England and Wales. J. chron. Dis. **15**, 85—90 (1962).

398. WYLIE, C. M.: (2) Late survival following cerebrovascular accidents. Arch. phys. Med. **43**, 297—300 (1962).
399. — Hospital care for patients with strokes in the acute stage. J. Amer. med. Ass. **193**, 791—795 (1965).
400. — (1) Do teaching hospitals provide better care for stroke? Physician's Panorama 4, 4—9 (1966).
401. — (2) Rehabilitative care of stroke patients. J. Amer. med. Ass. **196**, 1117—1120 (1966).
402. YANO, K., and S. UEDA: Coronary heart disease in Hiroshima, Japan: analysis of the data at the initial examination, 1958—1960. Yale J. Biol. Med. **35**, 504—522 (1963).
403. YATES, P. O.: A change in the pattern of cerebrovascular disease. Lancet **1964 I**, 65—69.
404. — The changing pattern of cerebrovascular disease in the United Kingdom. In: SIEKERT, R. G., and J. P. WHISNANT, Cerebral vascular diseases, pp. 67—82. New York: Grune and Stratton, 1966.
405. —, and E. C. HUTCHINSON: Cerebral infarction: The role of stenosis of the extracranial cerebral arteries. M.R.C. Special Report Series 300. London: H. M. Stationery Office, 1961.
406. YOSHITOSHI, Y. et. al.: Clinical features of myocardial infarction in Japan. Jap. Heart J. **5**, 497—511 (1964).
407. YOUNG, J. R., A. W. HUMPHRIES, V. G. DEWOLFE, E. G. BEVEN, and F. A. LeFEVRE: Extracranial cerebrovascular disease treated surgically, study of 100 patients. Arch. Surg. **89**, 848—855 (1964).
408. YULE, G. U., and M. G. KENDALL: An introduction to the theory of statistics, 14. Ed Revised and Enlarged. London: Charles Griffin & Co., 1950.
409. ZIELKE, H.-G., und K.-D. KRAFT: Statistische Untersuchungen an Patienten mit zerebralen Durchblutungsstörungen. Z. ges. inn. Med. **19**, 361—368 (1964).
410. ZSCHOCH, N.: Einige Bemerkungen zur statistischen Erfassung und Deutung von Sektionsbefunden. Zbl. allg. path. Anat. **100**, 80—83 (1959).
411. — Beitrag zur Todesursachenstatistik. Dtsch. Gesundh.-Wes. **19**, 311—314 (1964).
412. ZUMOFF, B., H. HART, and L. HELLMAN: Considerations of mortality in certain chronic diseases. Ann. intern. Med. **64**, 595—601 (1966).

Appendix

Table IV−a−1. *Age-specific annual mortality rates, cases per 100,000 population, for all cerebrovascular disease*

Age group	USA white 1960		USA white 1958		England-Wales 1960	
	M	F	M	F	M	F
< 1	—	—	4.9	3.7		
1— 4	—	—	1.1	0.7	0.7	0.5
5—14	—	—	0.7	0.6		
15—24	—	—	1.8	1.3	1.3	1.3
25—29	2.6	2.6	3.7	3.6		
30—34	4.3	4.1				
35—39	8.1	6.7	11.4	10.8	7.9	8.3
40—44	14.7	13.7				
45—49	28.7	25.3	42.4	35.5		
50—54	54.7	43.3			109	96
55—59	97.1	69.0	149.0	111.6		
60—64	189.1	141.6				
65—69	361.0	265.1	552.6	434.9	671	559
70—74	687.1	535.6				
75—79	1253.8	1092.0	1637.9	1494.0		
80—84	2195.1	2091.7			2146	2127
85 ≤	3734.8	3795.7	3639.2	4206.8		
Average	102.7 (BERKSON)	110.1	104.8 [WYLIE, 1962 (1)]	112.0	140 (DUBOULAY)	191

Table IV−a−2. *Cerebrovascular deaths in Denmark, 1950, by sex and age*

Age (years)	Male		Female		Total	
	pop. ×1000	No. CVD	pop. ×1000	No. CVD	pop. ×1000	No. CVD
0— 4	218.1	1	206.8	0	424.9	1
5—14	355.9	1	343.7	1	699.6	2
15—24	296.6	3	290.2	4	586.8	7
25—34	311.3	4	318.1	3	629.4	7
35—44	309.3	10	314.2	15	623.5	25
45—54	256.0	59	270.6	65	526.6	124
55—64	189.5	196	205.4	202	394.9	398
65—74	125.8	454	137.3	550	263.1	1004
75—84	49.2	543	56.7	659	105.9	1202
85 ≤	6.9	147	9.5	218	16.4	365
Total	2118.6	1418	2152.5	1717	4271.1	3135*

* 1467 died in hospital

Table IV−a−3. *Cerebrovascular deaths in Denmark,*
1950, as percent of total deaths, 1950, by age and sex

Age	Male	Female	Total
0— 4	0.06	0.00	0.03
5—14	0.52	0.76	0.62
15—24	1.02	2.27	1.49
25—34	0.86	0.85	0.85
35—44	1.33	2.19	1.74
45—54	3.70	4.52	4.09
55—64	6.66	8.16	7.34
65—74	9.16	11.46	10.29
75—84	10.57	11.44	11.03
85 ≤	7.97	9.13	8.62
Total	7.128	8.848	7.977

Table IV−a−4. *Cerebrovas-*
cular deaths in Sweden, 1956
to 1960, as percent of total
deaths by age and sex (Sta-
tistiska Centralbyrån 1966)

Age	Male	Female
0—	0.16	0.18
5—	0.71	0.64
10—	1.32	2.61
15—	1.60	1.49
20—	1.97	3.50
25—	2.22	2.74
30—	2.83	3.93
35—	3.94	4.98
40—	4.93	5.49
45—	6.18	9.54
50—	7.46	11.11
55—	8.08	12.95
60—	10.06	15.09
65—	12.29	17.44
70—	14.26	19.75
75—	16.18	20.07
80—	16.66	19.94
85—	15.51	17.24
90 ≤	12.84	13.26
Total	12.20	16.60

Table IV—a—5. *Cerebrovascular deaths in Denmark, 1950, age- and sex-specific mortality rates per 100,000 population*

Age	Male	Female	Total
0— 4	0.46	0	0.24
5—14	0.28	0.29	0.29
15—24	1.01	1.38	1.19
25—34	1.28	0.94	1.11
35—44	3.23	4.77	4.01
45—54	23.05	24.02	23.55
55—64	103.43	98.34	100.79
65—74	360.89	400.58	381.60
75—84	1103.66	1162.26	1135.03
85 ≤	2130.43	2294.74	2225.61
Total	66.93	79.76	73.40

Table IV—a—6. *Age- and sex-specific mortality rates for CVD deaths in Denmark, 1956, in cases per 100,000 population*

Age	Male			Female			Total		
	pop. ×1000	No. cases	rate	pop. ×1000	No. cases	rate	pop. ×1000	No. cases	rate
< 15	608.5	5	0.8	578.2	2	0.4	1184.7	7	0.6
15—24	304.3	3	1.0	297.9	3	1.0	602.2	6	1.0
25—34	293.6	2	0.7	300.5	3	1.0	594.1	5	0.8
35—44	306.3	17	5.6	311.8	17	5.5	618.1	34	5.5
45—54	283.5	67	23.6	293.5	93	31.7	577.0	160	27.7
55—64	213.2	238	111.6	233.3	255	109.3	446.5	493	110.4
65—74	138.5	673	485.9	156.0	788	505.1	294.5	1461	496.1
75—84	60.6	980	1617.2	68.3	1192	1745.2	128.9	2172	1685.0
85 ≤	8.8	359	4079.6	11.6	419	3612.1	20.4	778	3813.7
Total	2215.3	2344	105.8	2251.1	2771	123.1	4466.4	5115	114.5

Table IV—a—7. *Age- and sex-specific mortality rates for CVD deaths in Denmark, 1960, in cases per 100,000 population*

Age	Male			Female			Total		
	pop. ×1000	No. cases	rate	pop. ×1000	No. cases	rate	pop. ×1000	No. cases	rate
< 15	592.2	2	0.3	563.4	1	0.2	1155.6	3	0.3
15—24	348.1	4	1.2	335.9	1	0.3	684.0	5	0.7
25—34	280.8	3	1.1	284.9	10	3.5	565.7	13	2.3
35—44	301.8	10	3.3	309.3	15	4.9	611.1	25	4.1
45—54	295.1	60	20.3	303.2	61	20.1	598.3	121	20.2
55—64	230.3	241	104.7	251.4	210	83.5	481.7	451	93.6
65—74	147.2	682	463.3	169.6	730	430.2	316.8	1412	445.7
75—84	66.3	1040	1568.6	77.8	1350	1735.2	144.1	2390	1658.6
85 ≤	10.5	395	3761.9	13.2	510	3863.6	23.7	905	3818.6
Total	2272.3	2437	107.2	2308.7	2888	125.1	4581.0	5325	116.2

Table IV–a–8. *Age- and sex-specific mortality rates for CVD deaths in Norway, 1946, in cases per 100,000 population*

Age	Male			Female			Total		
	pop. ×1000	No. cases	rate	pop. ×1000	No. cases	rate	pop. ×1000	No. cases	rate
0— 9	261.3	5	1.9	248.1	3	1.2	509.4	8	1.6
10—19	215.6	2	0.9	207.6	1	0.5	423.2	3	0.7
20—29	273.1	7	2.6	267.6	0	0	540.8	7	1.3
30—39	246.8	8	3.2	248.7	7	2.8	495.4	15	3.0
40—49	200.4	34	17.0	218.6	36	16.5	419.0	70	16.7
50—59	154.4	83	53.8	170.2	123	72.3	324.7	206	63.4
60—69	103.8	248	238.9	122.9	288	234.3	226.7	536	236.4
70—79	60.3	432	716.4	75.1	573	763.0	135.4	1005	742.3
80—89	19.4	351	1809.3	27.7	488	1761.7	47.2	839	1777.5
90 ≤	1.6	54	3375.0	2.5	82	3280.0	4.1	136	3317.1
Total	1536.7	1224	79.7	1589.1	1621	102.0	3125.8	2845	91.0

Table IV–a–9. *Age- and sex-specific mortality rates for CVD deaths in Sweden, 1933, in cases per 100,000 population*

Age	Male			Female			Total		
	pop. ×1000	No. cases	rate	pop. ×1000	No. cases	rate	pop. ×1000	No. cases	rate
0—10	471.2	0	0	453.6	1	0.2	924.8	1	0.1
10—20	558.4	2	0.4	537.5	3	0.6	1095.9	5	0.5
20—30	547.3	10	1.8	538.8	10	1.9	1086.0	20	1.8
30—40	452.3	15	3.3	466.9	12	2.6	919.2	27	2.9
40—50	366.8	63	17.2	393.6	96	24.4	760.4	159	20.9
50—60	293.5	228	77.7	312.8	307	98.2	606.3	535	88.2
60—70	203.5	549	269.8	232.5	666	286.5	436.0	1215	278.7
70 ≤	106.5	1542	960.8	201.1	2027	1008.0	361.6	3569	987.0
Total	3053.5	2409	78.9	3136.8	3122	99.5	6190.4	5531	89.3

Table IV–a–10. *Age- and sex-specific mortality rates for CVD deaths in Sweden, 1960, in cases per 100,000 population*

Age	Male			Female			Total		
	pop. ×1000	No. cases	rate	pop. ×1000	No. cases	rate	pop. ×1000	No. cases	rate
0— 4	270.1	0	0	254.5	2	0.8	524.6	2	0.4
5—14	600.3	3	0.5	568.9	3	0.5	1169.3	6	0.5
15—24	513.9	7	1.4	497.5	3	0.6	1011.5	10	1.0
25—34	463.9	17	3.7	458.0	9	2.0	921.8	26	2.8
35—44	542.1	44	8.1	533.1	43	8.1	1075.2	87	8.1
45—54	529.0	164	31.0	525.9	156	29.7	1054.9	320	30.3
55—64	409.4	550	134.3	433.5	488	112.6	842.8	1038	123.2
65—74	262.6	1269	483.2	303.7	1497	492.9	566.3	2766	488.4
75—84	117.7	1859	1579.4	142.7	2393	1676.9	260.3	4250	1632.7
85 ≤	18.8	677	3601.1	25.8	894	3465.1	44.6	1571	3522.4
Total	3727.8	4590	123.1	3743.6	5486	146.5	7471.3	10076	134.9

Table IV−a−11. *Age- and sex-specific mortality rates for CVD deaths in Ireland, 1951, in cases per 100,000 population*

Age	Male			Female			Total		
	pop. ×1000	No. cases	rate	pop. ×1000	No. cases	rate	pop. ×1000	No. cases	rate
< 15	436.4	10	2.3	418.4	4	1.0	854.8	14	1.6
15—24	231.1	6	2.6	212.2	3	1.4	443.4	9	2.0
25—34	196.0	6	3.1	194.0	16	8.3	390.0	22	5.6
35—44	196.3	27	13.8	185.0	29	15.7	381.2	56	14.7
45—54	165.3	87	52.6	158.6	114	71.9	323.9	201	62.1
55—64	126.4	199	157.4	124.5	288	231.3	250.9	487	194.1
65—74	103.3	482	466.6	104.4	551	527.8	207.7	1033	497.4
75—84	46.3	476	1025.9	49.2	563	1144.3	95.4	1038	1088.1
85 ≤	5.5	68	1236.4	7.8	97	1243.6	13.3	165	1240.6
Total	1506.6	1360	90.3	1454.0	1665	114.5	2960.6	3025	102.2

Table IV−a−12. *Age- and sex-specific average annual mortality rates for cerebrovascular disease in Canada 1960—1964* (P. C. GORDON)

Age	Male	Female
20—24	1.9	1.7
25—29	2.3	2.3
30—34	3.8	3.7
35—39	7.2	6.8
40—44	11.6	11.0
45—49	23.6	24.6
50—54	45.3	46.5
55—59	85.4	78.6
60—64	172.8	141.2
65—69	311.8	254.5
70—74	608.9	536.6
75—79	1137.9	1060.7
80—84	1926.5	1982.7
85 ≤	3168.6	3684.9
Total	78.1	86.1
N	c. 7400	c. 7900

Table IV–a–13. *Age- and sex-specific average annual mortality rates, in cases per 100,000 population, for CVD deaths in San Francisco 1962—1964* (Sox)

Age	Male			Female			Total		
	pop. ×1000	av. No.*	rate	pop. ×1000	av. No.*	rate	pop. ×1000	av. No.*	rate
15—24	30.1	0	—	30.9	2.0	6.5	61.0	2.0	3.3
25—34	31.0	1.3	4.2	28.7	4.0	13.9	59.7	5.3	8.9
35—44	30.1	2.5	8.3	33.1	5.5	16.6	63.2	8.0	12.6
45—54	33.5	10.2	30.4	37.4	15.3	40.9	71.0	25.5	35.9
55—64	32.2	47.1	146.5	33.7	36.6	108.6	65.9	83.7	127.3
65—74	21.0	101.5	484.0	24.7	85.5	346.3	45.7	187.0	409.2
15—74	177.9	162.6	91.4	188.5	148.9	79.0	366.4	311.5	84.9

* weighted number of cases

Table IV–a–14. *Frequency distribution by sex and age groups in percentages for cerebrovascular disease, from population survey of Middlesex, Conn.*

Age	Male	Female	Total
< 35	0	1.0	0.5
35—44	0	1.0	0.5
45—54	6.6	5.0	5.8
55—64	18.7	14.0	16.2
65—74	34.1	23.0	28.3
75—84	30.8	30.0	30.4
85 ≤	9.9	26.0	18.3
Total	100.1	100.0	100.0
N	91	100	191

Table IV–a–15. *Age-specific incidence rates for all CVD from population surveys of Middlesex, Conn. and Rochester, Minn., in cases per 100,000 population, with 95% confidence limits on the rates*

Age	Middlesex		Rochester		Total		rate obs.	rate range
	No. cases	est. pop.*	No. cases	est. pop.*	No. cases	est. pop.*		
< 35	1	50,000	0	21,000	1	71,000	1.4	0.04–7.9
35—44	1	10,000	5	4,550	6	14,550	41.	15.1–89.8
45—54	11	10,000	6	4,000	17	14,000	121.	70.8–194.4
55—64	31	7,750	12	3,300	43	11,050	389.	281.6–524.3
65—74	54	5,740	14	2,400	68	8,140	835.	649. –1059.
75—84	58	2,650	19	1,150	77	3,800	2026.	1599. –2533.
85 ≤	35	690	8	288	43	978	4388.	3176. –5911.
Total	191	86,830	64	36,688	255	123,518	206.5	

* Population estimated from age-specific rates for each study.

Table IV–a–16. *Age-specific annual incidence rates, cases per 100,000 population for all cerebro-vascular disease from population surveys in USA*

age group	(1) Middlesex Conn.	(2) Rochester Minn.	(3) (1) + (2)*	(4) Du Pont Co.	(5) Chicago Ill.	(6) Framing-ham, Mass.	(7) New York a)	(8) b)
< 35	2	0	1					
35—39 / 40—44	10	110	40					
45—49 / 50—54	110	150	120	40 / 120	150	147	137	122
55—59 / 60—64	400	360	390	180 / 360				
65—69 / 70—74	940	580	840					
75—79 / 80—84	2190	1650	2060					
85 ≤	5070	2780	4400					
average	220 (170**)	174	207	—	—	—	—	—
N	191	64	255	?	9	90	108	51

* Weighted average
** Age-adjusted to US population
(1) EISENBERG; (2) KURLAND; (4) and (5) BERKSON; (6) KANNEL; (7) and (8) LADD

Table IV–a–17. *Age-specific annual incidence rates (cases per 100,000 pop.) for CVD in Carlisle, England 1955—1961 (BREWIS), and in three Missouri counties 1963—1964 (PARRISH), with 95% confidence limits on the rates*

Age	Population	N	rate	range
		A) Carlisle		
0—19	21,384	0	0.	0. — 17.3
20—29	8,492	7	11.8	0.3— 65.6
30—39	10,092	4	5.7	0.1— 47.6
40—49	9,681	27	39.8	10.5— 103.6
50—59	9,268	122	188.9	101. — 299.
60—69	7,297	220	429.9	294. — 610.
70—79	3,738	217	825.4	564. —1177.
80 ≤	1,149	97	1206.0	657. —2030.
	71,101	694	138.4	
		B) Missouri*		
< 35	—	0	0	
35—44	10,000	1	10	0— 56
45—54	7,790	7	90	36— 185
55—64	6,560	21	320	198— 490
65—74	5,420	52	960	717—1260
75—84	3,040	72	2370	1853—2984
85 ≤	750	42	5590	4025—7550
	—	195	258	

* Population estimated from cases and rates

Table IV−a−18. *Cerebrovascular disease in Goulburn, Australia, 1962—1964, percentage frequency by age and sex* (WALLACE)

Age	Male		Female		Total	
	N	%	N	%	N	%
0—39	3	5.1	5	5.8	8	5.5
40—49	3	5.1	8	9.3	11	7.6
50—59	6	10.2	10	11.6	16	11.0
60—69	15	25.4	22	25.6	37	25.5
70—79	18	30.5	25	29.1	43	29.7
80—89	11	18.6	14	16.3	25	17.2
90 ≤	3	5.1	2	2.3	5	3.5
Total	59	100.0	86	100.0	145	100.0

Table IV−a−19. *Annual incidence rates in cases per 100,000 population for cerebrovascular disease (330—334) in England and Wales, from 106 general practices* (LOGAN)

Age	Males		Females		Total			
	N*	rate	N*	rate	pop. ×1000	N	rate	range
0—14	0	0	0	0	83.3	0	0	0— 4
15—44	29	40	24	30	152.1	53	30	26— 46
45—64	199	430	196	370	99.2	395	400	360— 440
65 ≤	586	3040	828	2850	48.3	1414	2930	2780—3090
Total	804	450	1048	520	382.8	1862	490	

* N calculated from rates and populations for male and female by age group.

Table IV−a−20. *Cerebrovascular disease in Frederiksberg, Denmark, hospitalized cases only, 1940—1953, by age, sex, and average annual incidence rates in cases per 100,000 population, from material of* DALSGAARD-NIELSEN

Age	Σ Population	Male		Female		Total	
		No.	rate	No.	rate	No.	rate
< 50	79,634	29	5.9	30	5.2	59	5.5−
50—54	8,018	24	51.1	29	47.4	53	49.0
55—59	7,067	44	111.1	43	77.0	87	91.2
60—64	6,201	50	151.1	81	160.0	131	156.5−
65—69	5,157	74	269.6	93	220.7	167	239.9
70—74	3,585	77	421.5⁻	117	388.2	194	400.8
75—79	2,282	64	568.1	104	531.9	168	545.3
80—84	1,116	29	631.9	70	668.1	99	657.1
85 ≤	524	17	905.9	25	481.0	42	593.7
Total	113,584	408	60.7	592	68.9	1000	65.2
cases per annum		30.22		43.85		74.07	

Table IV – a – 21. *Sex Ratios in Cerebrovascular Disease. A. Total CVD. I — Mortality Statistics*

Source	Years	M/F (No. cases)	M/F (rates)	Median Age	N
Denmark	1950	0.83	0.84	74	3,135
Denmark	1956	0.85	0.86	76	5,115
Denmark	1960	0.84	0.86	76	5,325
Norway	1946	0.76	0.78	76	2,845
Sweden	1933	0.77	0.79	—	5,531
Sweden	1960	0.84	0.84	76	10,076
Eire	1951	0.82	0.79	73	3,025
US white (WYLIE, 1961)	1958	—	0.94	76	—
US white (BERKSON)	1960	0.91	0.93	—	169,053
US Negro (BERKSON)	1960	0.92	0.98	—	24,535
US white (BORHANI)	1949—1951	—	1.05	(35—64)	—
US white (BORHANI)	1959—1961	—	1.28	(35—64)	—
Surrey, England (CRAWFORD)	1962—1963	1.05	1.17	(45—59)	280
Carlisle, England (BREWIS)	1955—1961	—	1.03	—	—
San Francisco (SOX)	1962—1964	1.09	1.04	(15—74)	623

Table IV – a – 22. *Sex Ratios in Cerebrovascular Disease. A. Total CVD. II — Other Statistics*

Source	Years	M/F (No. cases)	M/F (rates)	Median Age	N
IIa. Hospital Series					
Saskatchewan (WYLIE)	1959—1963	1.23	1.16	74	10,701
Belfast (ADAMS)	1948—1956	0.79	—	69	710
London (MARSHALL)	1950—1954	1.76	—	59	251
Leipzig (ZIELKE)	1953—1961	0.82	—	68	2,009
Vienna (FELGER)	1951—1955	1.25	—	63	1,000
Florence, Venice, Trieste (FUMAGALLI)	1951—1953	0.95	—	67	2,178
Fredericksberg, Denmark (DALSGAARD)	1940—1953	0.69	0.88	70	1,000
Hyderabad, India (NAIK)	1961—1963	1.75*	—	c. 53	866
IIb. Population Surveys					
Framingham, Mass. (KANNEL)	1949—1962	0.84	—	—	90
Rochester, Minn. (KURLAND)	1957	1.06	1.37	66	64
Middlesex, Conn. (EISENBERG)	1957—1958	0.91	0.92	73	191
mid-Missouri (PARRISH)	1963—1964	0.79	0.89	c. 77	195
Goulburn, Australia (WALLACE)	1962—1964	0.72	—	70	155
England-Wales (LOGAN)	1955—1956	0.77	0.87	<65	c. 1,862

* Ratio for all patients = 1.63

Table V−a−1. *Distribution of cerebrovascular deaths in Norway,*
1946

No.	Area	pop. ×1000	No. cases	% mean rate
1.	Ostfold	178.4	191	123.27
2.	Akershus	587.3	503	98.61
3.	Hedmark	169.5	168	114.12
4.	Opland	154.7	114	84.84
5.	Buskerud	149.9	144	110.60
6.	Vestfold	147.6	144	112.33
7.	Telemark	131.7	109	95.29
8.	Aust Agder	74.9	85	130.66
9.	Vest Agder	94.0	94	115.13
10.	Rogaland	202.3	126	71.71
11.	Hordaland	298.8	208	80.15
12.	Sogn og Fjordane	96.8	99	117.75
13.	Møre og Romsdal	182.9	166	104.50
14.	Sør Trøndelag	193.9	186	110.44
15.	Nord Trøndelag	105.7	110	119.82
16.	Nordland	216.0	167	89.02
17.	Troms	113.7	82	83.04
18.	Finmark	58.8	46	90.07
Total		3157.0	2742	100.00 =
		$\chi^2 = 64.47$		86.8546
				per 100,000

Table V−a−2. *Distribution of CVD deaths in Norway, 1946, with*
population 60 or older as base

No.	Area	Population	No. CVD	% mean rate
1.	Ostfold	23,763	191	122.66
2.	Akershus	75,296	503	101.94
3.	Hedmark	22,485	168	114.02
4.	Opland	20,686	114	84.10
5.	Buskerud	21,579	144	101.83
6.	Vestfold	20,533	144	107.02
7.	Telemark	19,235	109	86.48
8.	Aust Adger	12,534	85	103.49
9.	Vest Adger	13,914	94	103.09
10.	Rogaland	24,928	126	77.13
11.	Hordaland	39,275	208	80.82
12.	Sogn og Fjordane	15,323	99	98.59
13.	Møre og Romsdal	25,625	166	98.86
14.	Sør Trøndelag	25,609	186	110.84
15.	Nord Trøndelag	14,040	110	119.56
16.	Nordland	25,886	167	89.45—
17.	Troms	12,586	82	99.42
18.	Finmark	5,169	46	135.80
Total		418,466	2742	100.00 =
		$\chi^2 = 45.64$		65.525
				per 10,000

Table V–a–3. *Distributions in Norway. II. Physicians in 1946*

No.	Area	1946 MD	MD prev.*	prev. rank	χ^2_a rank
1.	Ostfold	113	63.34	8	6
2.	Akershus	1015	172.83	1	1
3.	Hedmark	96	56.64	10	10
4.	Opland	83	53.65	11	13
5.	Buskerud	107	71.38	5	5
6.	Vestfold	78	52.85	12	15
7.	Telemark	95	72.13	4	4
8.	Aust Agder	63	84.11	2	2
9.	Vest Agder	73	77.60	3	3
10.	Rogaland	124	61.30	9	8
11.	Hordaland	191	63.92	6	9
12.	Sogn og Fjordane	42	43.39	16	16
13.	Møre og Romsdal	76	41.55	17	17
14.	Sør Trøndelag	123	63.44	7	7
15.	Nord Trøndelag	52	49.20	14	11
16.	Nordland	95	43.98	15	18
17.	Troms	57	50.13	13	12
18.	Finmark	22	37.42	18	14
Total		2505	79.348		

* MD prev. = No. MD/100,000 population, rounded

Table V−a−4. Distributions in Norway. III. Summary of hospital data 1946 and 1948

No.	Area	Hospitals 1946			Hospitals 1948			Genl Hosp. 1948			Hospital beds 1946			Hospital Adm. 1946			Hosp. beds 1948		
		No.	rank	prev. χ_a^2	No.	rank	prev. χ_a^2	No.	rank	prev. χ_a^2	No.	rank	prev. χ_a^2	No.	rank	prev. χ_a^2	No.	rank	prev. χ_a^2
1.	Ostfold	13	10	9	13	9	9	4	8	8	633	13	14	11022	13	14	625	14	15
2.	Akershus	22	17	18	22	18	18	14	6	6	5019	1	1	76856	1	1	5415	1	1
3.	Hedmark	18	3	3	19	2	3	3	13	14	596	14	2	11739	10	12	735	12	11
4.	Opland	10	12	12	10	11	11	3	11	11	438	16	17	3933	18	18	490	16	16
5.	Buskerud	5	18	17	6	17	16	2	18	17	492	15	15	11788	7	7	519	15	14
6.	Vestfold	7	14	13	7	14	13	4	5	5	537	12	12	10194	11	10	518	13	13
7.	Telemark	13	4	4	13	4	4	4	4	4	593	8	9	9940	8	8	595	9	9
8.	Aust Agder	6	6	7	6	8	8	1	17	15	360	5	6	5933	6	6	350	8	8
9.	Vest Agder	7	9	10	8	6	6	4	2	2	415	9	10	8650	4	4	457	7	6
10.	Rogaland	10	13	14	10	13	14	4	10	12	1013	4	5	18859	2	2	1063	5	5
11.	Hordaland	13	16	16	13	16	17	4	16	18	1183	10	13	22122	9	9	1349	10	12
12.	Sogn of Fjordane	8	5	5	8	7	7	4	3	3	270	17	16	4363	17	16	252	18	17
13.	Møre og Romsdal	8	15	15	8	15	15	3	15	16	498	18	18	10383	15	15	515	17	18
14.	Sør Trøndelag	13	11	11	13	10	10	4	9	9	1021	3	4	18048	3	3	1070	4	3
15.	Nord Trøndelag	8	8	8	6	12	12	2	12	10	484	7	8	9293	5	5	589	3	4
16.	Nordland	25	2	2	24	3	2	5	7	7	838	11	11	10675	16	17	965	11	10
17.	Troms	9	7	6	11	5	5	2	14	13	532	6	7	7307	12	13	555	6	7
18.	Finmark	12	1	1	19	1	1	4	1	1	358	2	3	3626	14	11	440	2	2
	Total	207	6.557	= prev.	216	6.842	= prev.	71	2.249	= prev.	15280	484.00	= prev.	254731 8069.		= prev.	16502	522.71	= prev.

154 Appendix

Table V–a–5. *Distributions of urban CVD deaths in Sweden 1933, with urban population 60 or older as base*

No.	Area	Population	No. CVD	% mean rate
1.	Stockholm	60,387	299	82.62
1.a	Stockholmslän	6,309	44	116.37
2.	Upsala	5,552	26	78.14
3.	Södermanlands	8,743	68	129.78
4.	Östergöttlands	16,078	114	118.31
5.	Jönköpings	8,662	62	119.43
6.	Kronobergs	1,329	10	125.55
7.	Kalmar	6,567	34	86.39
8.	Gottlands	1,559	13	139.14
9.	Blekinge	5,460	50	152.80
10.	Kristianstads	3,052	24	131.21
11.	Malmohus	31,761	169	88.79
12.	Hallands	5,811	28	80.40
13.	Göteborg-Bohus	31,731	132	69.41
14.	Älvsborgs	9,178	64	116.36
15.	Skaraborgs	6,687	45	112.89
16.	Värmlands	6,437	47	121.83
17.	Örebro	6,279	46	122.24
18.	Västmanlands	7,139	40	93.49
19.	Kopparbergs	3,282	21	106.77
20.	Gävleborgs	7,272	63	144.56
21.	Västernorrlands	4,068	43	176.38
22.	Jämtlands	1,478	12	135.48
23.	Västerbottens	1,327	15	188.61
24.	Norbottens	2,473	21	141.69
Total		248,621	1490	100.00=

$$\chi^2 = 97.34$$

59.931

per 10,000

Table V−a−6. *Distribution by county of deaths due to CVD in Sweden. 1960*

No.	Area	pop. ×1000	No. cases	% mean rate
1.	Stockholm	807.9	846	77.7
1.a	Stockholmslän	446.1	484	80.5
2.	Upsala	166.8	164	72.9
3.	Södermanlands	225.9	339	111.3
4.	Östergöttlands	358.5	480	99.3
5.	Jönköpings	284.0	391	102.1
6.	Kronobergs	159.3	237	110.3
7.	Kalmar	236.6	366	114.7
8.	Gottlands	55.1	84	113.0
9.	Blekinge	144.6	200	102.6
10.	Kristianstads	257.3	368	106.1
11.	Malmöhus	622.1	804	95.8
12.	Hallands	169.4	273	119.5
13.	Göteborgs-Bohus	619.7	717	85.8
14.	Älvsborgs	373.7	499	99.0
15.	Skaraborgs	249.7	454	134.8
16.	Värmlands	291.2	529	134.7
17.	Örebro	261.4	437	124.0
18.	Västmanlands	230.0	261	84.2
19.	Kopparbergs	286.2	411	106.5
20.	Gävleborgs	294.0	418	105.4
21.	Västernorrlands	288.2	497	127.9
22.	Jämtlands	141.4	228	119.6
23.	Västerbottens	240.4	293	90.4
24.	Norbottens	261.9	296	83.8
Total		7471.3	10,076	100.00=

$$\chi^2 = 305.63$$

134.863 per 100,000

Appendix

Table V–a–7. *Distribution of CVD deaths in Sweden 1960, with*
population 60 or older as base

No.	Area	popu-lation	No. CVD	rate per 10 M	% mean rate
1.	Stockholm	140,361	846	60.27	77.38
1.a	Stockholmslän	62,134	484	77.90	100.01
2.	Upsala	30,708	164	53.41	68.57
3.	Södermanlands	40,289	339	84.14	108.03
4.	Östergöttlands	63,367	480	75.75⁻	97.25
5.	Jönköpings	49,549	391	78.91	101.31
6.	Kronobergs	31,538	237	75.15⁻	96.48
7.	Kalmar	44,427	366	82.38	105.77
8.	Gottlands	10,118	84	83.02	106.59
9.	Blekinge	27,318	200	73.21	93.99
10.	Kristianstads	50,323	368	73.13	93.89
11.	Malmöhus	112,572	804	71.42	91.69
12.	Hallands	31,524	273	86.60	111.18
13.	Göteborgs-Bohus	103,479	717	69.29	88.96
14.	Älvsborgs	67,364	499	74.08	95.10
15.	Skaraborgs	48,540	454	93.53	120.08
16.	Värmlands	53,951	529	98.05	125.89
17.	Örebro	47,125	437	92.73	119.06
18.	Västmanlands	34,944	261	74.69	95.89
19.	Kopparbergs	51,097	411	80.44	103.27
20.	Gävleborgs	53,446	418	78.21	100.41
21.	Västernorrlands	49,027	497	101.37	130.15⁻
22.	Jämtlands	25,784	228	88.43	113.53
23.	Västerbottens	33,900	293	86.43	110.96
24.	Norbottens	30,792	296	96.13	123.42
Total		1,293,677	10,076		100.00=

$$\chi^2 = 218.59$$

77.887
per 10,000

Table V–a–8. Distributions in Sweden. II. Summary of Physicians and Hospitals, 1933

No.	Area	Physicians			Hospitals			Hospital beds			Hospital Admissions		
		No.	rank prev.	χ^2_a	No.	rank prev.	χ^2_a	No.	rank prev.	χ^2_a	No.	rank prev.	χ^2_a
1.	Stockholm	755	1	1	8	11	11	3839	1	1	38259	1	1
1.a	Stockholmslän	107	5	5	6	2	2	734	8	8	12735	7	7
2.	Upsala	89	2	2	1	24	23	636	2	3	9765	2	3
3.	Södermanlands	67	6	7	4	3	3	535	7	7	9516	5	5
4.	Östergöttlands	106	8	9	6	7	5	1055	4	4	13856	8	8
5.	Jönköpings	62	18	19	3	18	18	463	19	19	8764	16	16
6.	Kronobergs	33	25	22	2	19	17	230	24	23	4365	25	24
7.	Kalmar	63	17	18	4	10	9	408	22	22	7557	23	22
8.	Gottlands	13	23	10	1	9	10	95	23	15	2079	18	12
9.	Blekinge	43	12	11	2	16	16	306	17	16	6133	10	9
10.	Kristianstads	62	20	23	3	21	21	560	15	17	9572	13	15
11.	Malmöhus	260	3	3	7	17	19	2337	3	2	33393	3	2
12.	Hallands	49	9	8	3	6	7	371	11	12	6282	11	10
13.	Göteborgs-Bohus	212	4	4	7	12	12	1255	9	9	17050	17	20
14.	Älvsborgs	97	10	14	3	23	24	582	20	24	10590	22	23
15.	Skaraborgs	72	11	12	3	20	20	595	12	13	10304	9	11
16.	Värmlands	75	16	21	4	14	14	550	18	20	9301	21	21
17.	Örebro	62	15	15	1	25	25	400	21	21	7881	19	18
18.	Västmanlands	43	19	13	4	1	1	540	5	5	8093	6	6
19.	Kopparbergs	72	14	16	5	4	4	540	16	18	9490	15	17
20.	Gävleborgs	65	22	25	4	15	15	677	14	14	10005	20	19
21.	Västernorrlands	82	13	17	5	8	8	820	6	6	14200	4	4
22.	Jämtlands	46	7	6	2	13	13	330	13	11	5126	14	13
23.	Västerbottens	44	24	24	2	22	22	527	10	10	7995	12	14
24.	Norbottens	50	21	20	4	5	6	252	25	25	5747	24	25
Total		2629	100.0% = 42.788 prev.		94	100.00% = 1.530 prev.		18637	100.00% = 303.33 prev.		278058	100.00% = 4525. prev.	

Table V–a–9. *Distribution in Sweden. III. Urban practicing physicans, 1933*

No.	Area	urban population 1935	No. MD	% mean prev.	prev. rank	χ^2_a rank
1.	Stockholm	534,236	700	154.26	4	1
1.a	Stockholmslän	51,519	31	70.84	20	16
2.	Upsala	39,894	60	177.06	2	2
3.	Södermanlands	64,969	40	72.48	18	18
4.	Östergöttlands	115,849	76	77.23	16	20
5.	Jönköpings	75,171	38	59.51	24	24
6.	Kronobergs	9,835	15	179.56	1	3
7.	Kalmar	52,247	34	76.61	17	15
8.	Gottlands	11,141	9	95.11	9	8
9.	Blekinge	46,486	33	83.58	15	13
10.	Kristianstads	26,267	29	129.98	5	5
11.	Malmöhus	277,426	204	86.57	11	19
12.	Hallands	46,262	34	86.53	12	11
13.	Göteborg-Bohus	304,259	174	67.33	22	25
14.	Älvsborgs	88,347	53	70.63	21	22
15.	Skaraborgs	51,210	42	96.56	8	9
16.	Värmlands	52,322	38	85.50	13	12
17.	Örebro	47,791	34	83.76	14	14
18.	Västmanlands	51,798	29	65.91	23	21
19.	Kopparbergs	30,760	23	88.03	10	10
20.	Gävleborgs	58,107	35	70.91	19	17
21.	Västernorrlands	38,977	38	114.78	6	6
22.	Jämtlands	15,077	20	156.17	3	4
23.	Västerbottens	20,624	18	102.75	7	7
24.	Norbottens	26,278	8	35.84	25	23
Total		2,136,852	1815	100.00 = 84.938		

Table V−a−10. *Distribution of deaths due to "CVD"* in Denmark,*
1950

No.	Area	pop. ×1000	No. cases	% mean rate
1.+2.	Copenhagen + Roskilde	1263.5	981	89.12
3.	Frederiksborg	146.9	140	109.39
4.	Holbaek	126.8	99	89.62
5.	Sorø	126.2	123	111.87
6.	Praestø	123.4	94	87.44
7.	Bornholms	48.6	61	144.07
8.	Maribo	136.2	144	121.36
9.	Svendborg	150.0	129	98.71
10.	Odense	245.2	230	107.67
11.	Vejle	201.3	205	116.89
12.	Skanderborg	133.8	142	121.82
13.	Aarhus	196.7	184	107.37
14.	Randers	167.9	145	99.13
15.	Aalborg	225.8	191	97.09
16.	Hjørring	169.9	133	89.85
17.	Thisted	88.4	107	138.94
18.	Viborg	156.9	135	98.76
19.	Ringkøbing	187.2	145	88.91
20.	Ribe	170.2	137	92.39
21.	Haderslev	69.8	65	106.89
22.	Aabenraa-Sønderborg	94.1	98	119.54
23.	Tønder	42.3	33	89.55
Total		4271.1	3721	100.00=
		$\chi^2 = 65.08$		87.1204 per 100,000

* Neurologic deaths, 85% = CVD (same rate for capital, urban and rural, and Copenhagen hospital deaths)

Appendix

Table V-a-11. *Denmark. Distribution of "CVD"* deaths by county, 1950, against population age 60 or more*

No.	Area	pop. 60 ≤	No. "CVD"*	% mean rate
1.	Copenhagen area	161,692	932	88.68
2.	Roskilde	10,527	49	71.61
	(1. + 2.)	(172,219)	(981)	(89.12)
3.	Frederiksborg	19,692	140	109.38
4.	Holbaek	18,872	99	80.71
5.	Sorø	18,213	123	103.90
6.	Praestø	18,716	94	77.27
7.	Bornholms	7,112	61	131.95
8.	Maribo	20,725	144	106.89
9.	Svendborg	24,152	129	82.17
10.	Odense	33,377	230	106.01
11.	Vejle	26,790	205	117.72
12.	Skanderborg	18,593	142	117.50
13.	Aarhus	25,420	184	111.36
14.	Randers	22,269	145	100.17
15.	Aalborg	26,099	191	112.59
16.	Hjørring	20,759	133	98.57
17.	Thisted	11,858	107	138.82
18.	Viborg	19,703	135	105.41
19.	Ringkøbing	20,939	145	106.54
20.	Ribe	19,984	137	105.47
21.	Haderslev	9,173	65	109.02
22.	Aabenraa-Sönderborg	12,479	98	120.82
23.	Tønder	5,315	33	95.52
Total		572,459	3721	100.00=
		$\chi^2 = 73.33$		65.000 per 10,000

* Neurologic deaths, 85% CVD

Table V–a–12. Distributions in Denmark. II. Summary of physicians 1950

No.	Area	1950 pop. ×1000	All MD 1950 No.	rank prev.	χ^2_a	Settled MD No.	rank prev.	Younger MD No.	rank prev.	Neural Specialists No.	rank prev.	χ^2_a
1.	Copenhagen area	1187.1										
2.	Roskilde	76.4										
1.+2.		(1263.5)	(1960)	(1)	(1)	(1144)	(1)	(816)	(1)	(216)	(1)	(1)
3.	Frederiksborg	146.9	150	3	3	110	3	40	4	8	11	11
4.	Holbaek	126.8	120	5	5	82	7	38	3	9	7	7
5.	Sorø	126.2	99	12	11	77	11	22	15	6	13	12
6.	Praestø	123.4	115	6	6	85	5	30	8	9	6	5
7.	Bornholms	48.6	30	19	15	26	18	4	21	1	20	13
8.	Maribo	136.2	97	16	18	84	10	13	20	8	10	10
9.	Svendborg	150.0	124	10	8	95	8	29	11	5	15	19
10.	Odense	245.2	210	8	12	147	12	63	6	19	4	6
11.	Vejle	201.3	169	9	10	118	15	51	7	14	9	9
12.	Skanderborg	133.8	121	7	7	93	4	28	9	10	5	4
13.	Aarhus	196.7	267	2	2	150	2	117	2	31	2	2
14.	Randers	167.9	137	11	13	106	9	31	13	4	18	21
15.	Aalborg	225.8	163	15	21	121	17	42	12	11	12	17
16.	Hjørring	169.9	115	18	20	88	20	27	16	2	21	22
17.	Thisted	88.4	52	21	19	40	22	12	17	2	19	18
18.	Viborg	156.9	120	14	16	88	16	32	10	11	8	8
19.	Ringkøbing	187.2	110	22	22	87	21	23	18	6	16	20
20.	Ribe	170.2	132	13	17	101	13	31	14	8	14	15
21.	Haderslev	69.8	49	17	9	41	14	8	19	2	17	14
22.	Aabenraa-Sønderborg	94.1	89	4	4	64	6	25	5	10	3	3
23.	Tønder	42.3	25	20	14	22	19	3	22	0	22	16
Total		4271.1	4454	104.2 av. prev.		2969	69.6 av. prev.	1485	34.8 av. prev.	392	9.17 av. prev.	

Table V – a – 13. Distributions in Denmark. III. Summary of neural specialists 1950 and general hospitals 1950

No.	Area	Neurologists No.	rank prev.	χ²a	Internists No.	rank prev.	χ²a	Ophthalmologists No.	rank prev.	χ²a	No. General Hosp. No.	rank prev.	χ²a	No. Gen. Hosp. beds No.	rank prev.	χ²a
1.+2.	Copenhagen area	(39)	(2)	(1)	(119)	(1)	(1)	(35)	(1)	(1)	22	23	23	9049	2	1
2.	Roskilde	4	4	4	3	15	16	—	21.5	22	3	15	19	505	3	3
3.	Frederiksborg	4	1	3	3	11	10	1	17	17	6	13	12	716	13	14
4.	Holbaek	—	16.5	17	3	10	9	1	16	16	6	8	9	616	14	12
5.	Sorø										7	3	4	668	10	10
6.	Praestø	1	8	8	3	9	8	2	7	7	6	7	7	646	11	11
7.	Bornholms	—	16.5	10	—	21.5	15	1	3	6	5	1	1	284	7	6
8.	Maribo	2	5	5	4	7	7	2	8	9	7	6	5	529	22	23
9.	Svendborg	—	16.5	19	3	16	17	2	10	10	7	10	8	952	4	4
10.	Odense	3	6	6	9	6	6	3	12	14	8	20	20	1089	19	22
11.	Vejle	1	10	14	8	5	5	4	5	4	8	14	14	1180	6	7
12.	Skanderborg	—	16.5	18	7	4	4	3	2	2	6	11	10	727	9	9
13.	Aarhus	6	3	2	16	2	2	4	4	3	7	17	17	1687	1	2
14.	Randers	—	16.5	20.5	3	17	21	1	18	19	6	16	15	806	15	16
15.	Aalborg	1	11	16	5	13	20	3	11	12	8	18	17	1061	16	19
16.	Hjørring	—	16.5	20.5	1	20	22	1	19	20	9	5	3	829	12	15
17.	Thisted	—	16.5	13	1	19	18	1	13	11	6	2	2	366	21	18
18.	Viborg	1	9	11	4	8	12	3	6	5	3	22	22	873	8	8
19.	Ringkøbing	—	16.5	22	4	14	19	2	14	15	5	21	21	851	17	20
20.	Ribe	2	7	7	4	12	14	1	20	21	6	19	17	757	18	21
21.	Haderslev	—	16.5	12	1	18	11	1	9	8	3	12	13	308	20	13
22.	Aabenraa-Sønderborg	—	16.5	15	6	3	3	1	15	13	5	4	6	582	5	5
23.	Tønder	—	16.5	9	—	21.5	13	—	21.5	18	2	9	11	144	23	17
	Total	64	1.498 av. prev.		207	4.846 av. prev.		72	1.686 av. prev.		151	3.535 av. prev.		25225	590.61 av. prev.	

Table V–a–14. *Distribution by county of deaths due to CVD in Denmark, 1960*

No.	Area	pop. ×1000	No. cases	% mean rate
1.	Copenhagen	1321.5	1264	82.3
2.	Roskilde	89.8	106	101.6
3.	Frederiksborg	180.1	196	93.6
4.	Holbaek	127.1	143	96.8
5.	Sorø	129.8	175	116.0
6.	Praestø	122.1	170	119.8
7.	Bornholms	48.5	68	120.7
8.	Maribo	132.3	201	130.7
9.	Svendborg	149.1	204	117.7
10.	Odense	264.4	402	130.8
11.	Vejle	213.8	290	116.7
12.	Skanderborg	138.0	222	138.4
13.	Aarhus	220.2	241	94.2
14.	Randers	170.0	186	94.1
15.	Aalborg	238.8	257	92.6
16.	Hjørring	177.6	224	108.5
17.	Thisted	85.1	107	108.2
18.	Viborg	161.9	191	101.5
19.	Ringkøbing	205.4	215	90.1
20.	Ribe	184.9	211	98.2
21.	Haderslev	72.5	71	84.3
22.	Aabenraa-Sønderborg	105.6	125	101.8
23.	Tønder	42.5	56	113.4
Total		4581.0	5325	100.00=

$$\chi^2 = 151.41 \qquad \begin{matrix} 116.241 \\ \text{per } 100{,}000 \end{matrix}$$

11*

Appendix

Table V – a – 15. *Denmark. Distribution of CVD deaths by county,*
1960, against population age 60 or more

No.	area	pop. 60 ≤	No. CVD	% mean rate
1.	Copenhagen	209,226	1264	80.83
2.	Roskilde	13,253	106	107.01
	(1. + 2.)	(222,479)	(1370)	(82.39)
3.	Frederiksborg	24,775	196	105.85⁻
4.	Holbaek	22,337	143	85.66
5.	Sorø	21,751	175	107.65⁻
6.	Praestø	21,276	170	106.91
7.	Bornholms	8,117	68	112.09
8.	Maribo	24,125	201	111.47
9.	Svendborg	27,581	204	98.96
10.	Odense	40,936	402	131.39
11.	Vejle	32,932	290	117.82
12.	Skanderborg	22,836	222	130.07
13.	Aarhus	33,062	241	97.53
14.	Randers	27,363	186	90.95⁻
15.	Aalborg	33,879	257	101.50
16.	Hjørring	25,997	224	115.28
17.	Thisted	14,095	107	101.60
18.	Viborg	24,431	191	104.60
19.	Ringkøbing	26,646	215	107.96
20.	Ribe	25,227	211	111.91
21.	Handerslev	10,802	71	87.94
22.	Aabenraa-Sønderborg	15,219	125	109.89
23.	Tønder	6,580	56	113.87
Total		712,446	5325	100.00=
		$\chi^2 = 134.41$		74.743 per 10,000

Table V−a−16. *Percentage frequency distribution of CVD deaths in Denmark, 1960, by age, sex, and area*

Sex and age	Capital			Provincial Towns	Rural	Total
	Copenhagen	Fredericks-berg	Gentofte			
			Male			
< 35	0.31	0	0	0.43	0.39	0.37
35—44	0.63	0	0	0	0.63	0.41
45—64	18.50	12.70	9.86	12.64	10.78	12.35
65—84	71.47	76.19	69.01	70.88	70.16	70.66
85 ≤	9.09	11.11	21.13	16.05	18.05	16.21
100.00% =	319	63	71	704	1280	2437
			Female			
< 35	0	0	1.14	0.57	0.44	0.41
35—44	1.16	0.85	0	0.79	0.15	0.52
45—64	11.57	12.82	5.68	8.39	9.28	9.38
65—84	71.99	64.96	71.59	73.02	72.02	72.02
85 ≤	15.28	21.37	21.59	17.23	18.12	17.66
100.00% =	432	117	88	882	1369	2888
			Total			
< 35	0.13	0	0.63	0.50	0.42	0.39
35—44	0.93	0.56	0	0.44	0.38	0.47
45—64	14.51	12.78	7.55	10.28	10.00	10.74
65—84	71.77	68.89	70.44	72.07	71.12	71.40
85 ≤	12.65	17.78	21.38	16.71	18.08	17.00
100.00% =	751	180	159	1586	2649	5325

Table V−a−17. *Some correlations of distributions by county of medical facilities in Sweden, 1933*

Factors	r	t
hospital beds vs. admissions	+0.90	+10.18
hospital beds vs. number of hospitals	+0.20	+ 0.96
hospital beds vs. population density	+0.49	+ 2.70
hospitals beds vs. all physicians	+0.68	+ 4.44
hospital beds vs. urban physicians	+0.19	—
physicians vs. population density	+0.62	+ 3.79
physicians vs. number of hospitals	+0.11	—
physicians vs. urban physicians	+0.09	—
urban physicians vs. number of hospitals	—0.35	— 1.76
urban physicians vs. hospital beds	+0.19	—
urban physicians vs. hospitals admissions	+0.27	—
urban physicians vs. population density	—0.05	—

P = 0.05 r = +0.34, t = ±2.07
P = 0.01 r = +0.48, t = ±2.50

Table V−a−18. *Distribution of cerebrovascular disease in Ireland: percent of average annual mortality rate (1951—1955) by county recalculated from* ACHESON *(1960):*

No.	County	Male	Female	Total
1.	Carlow	100.0	70.4	82.2
2.	Cavan	100.0	117.7	107.9
3.	Clare	79.1	79.2	78.4
4. + 28.	Cork, Cork C. B.	109.3	107.2	109.8*
5.	Donegal	115.9	99.6	106.2
6.+29.+30.	Dublin, Dublin C. B. Dun Laoghaire C. B.	114.2*	103.2	107.3*
7.	Galway	84.1	83.2	82.7
8.	Kerry	80.8	89.8	84.7
9.	Kildare	71.4	95.6	82.6
10.	Kilkenny	88.5	85.8	85.7
11.	Laoighis	104.9	118.6	110.3
12.	Leitrim	109.3	114.6	110.7
13.+31.	Limerick, Lim. C. B.	72.6	75.2	73.0
14.	Longford	64.3	47.3	54.9
15.	Louth	101.1	112.4	106.8
16.	Mayo	60.4	58.4	58.9
17.	Meath	106.6	107.5	106.0
18.	Monaghan	86.3	112.4	99.2
19.	Offaly	95.1	107.5	100.2
20.	Roscommon	78.0	80.5	78.6
21.	Sligo	104.9	85.0	93.5
22.	Tipperary, N.R.	114.3	98.7	105.0
23.	Tipperary, S. R.	119.8	115.0	116.2
24.+32.	Waterford, Wat. C. B.	101.2	125.7*	113.8
25.	Westmeath	101.6	124.3	116.7
26.	Wexford	133.0*	134.1**	132.8**
27.	Wicklow	168.7**	163.3**	164.7**
		100.0 = 78.3	100.0 = 97.2	100.0 = 88.0
		N = 1182.0 (78.5)	1419.0 (97.6)	2601.0 (87.8)
		$\chi^2 = 48.84$	54.66	96.81

Table V−a−19. *Non-federal physicians in the United States, 1962*

No.	State	pop. ×1000	MD	% mean rate
1.	Maine	978	1,198	90.7
2.	New Hampshire	622	858	102.1
3.	Vermont	387	637	121.9
4.	Massachusetts	5,188	9,746	139.1
5.	Connecticut	2,625	4,520	127.5
6.	Rhode Island	878	1,231	103.8
7.	New York	17,498	34,274	145.0
8.	New Jersey	6,357	8,470	98.7
9.	Pennsylvania	11,382	16,752	109.0
10.	Ohio	10,038	13,112	96.7
11.	Indiana	4,663	4,873	77.4
12.	Illinois	10,098	13,586	99.6
13.	Michigan	8,029	10,884	100.4
14.	Wisconsin	4,019	4,530	83.5⁻
15.	Minnesota	3,461	4,918	105.2
16.	Iowa	2,774	3,257	86.9
17.	Missouri	4,316	6,259	107.4
18.	North Dakota	633	534	62.5⁻
19.	South Dakota	721	536	55.1
20.	Nebraska	1,446	1,598	81.8
21.	Kansas	2,215	2,484	83.0
22.	Delaware	467	586	92.9
23.	Maryland	3,233	4,648	106.5⁻
24.	Virginia	4,248	4,312	75.2
24.a	Washington, D. C.	789	2,705	253.9
25.	W. Virginia	1,796	1,801	74.3
26.	N. Carolina	4,704	4,412	69.5⁻
27.	S. Carolina	2,448	1,848	55.9
28.	Georgia	4,083	3,843	69.7
29.	Florida	5,434	7,159	97.6
30.	Kentucky	3,084	2,806	67.4
31.	Tennessee	3,652	4,014	81.4
32.	Alabama	3,317	2,518	56.2
33.	Mississippi	2,261	1,685	55.2
34.	Arkansas	1,842	1,583	63.6
35.	Louisiana	3,371	3,708	81.5⁻
36.	Oklahoma	2,448	2,732	82.6
37.	Texas	10,122	10,715	78.4
38.	Montana	697	692	73.5
39.	Idaho	700	631	66.8
40.	Wyoming	332	313	69.8
41.	Colorado	1,893	3,008	117.7
42.	New Mexico	997	880	65.4
43.	Arizona	1,486	1,675	83.5⁻
44.	Utah	958	1,181	91.3
45.	Nevada	350	335	70.9
46.	Washington	3,010	4,028	99.1
47.	Oregon	1,807	2,569	105.3
48.	California	5,517	29,020	126.2
Total		184,886	249,664	100.00= 135.037

Table V–a–20. *CVD distribution in Denmark by age-group for residence in nine areas: population (1960) vs. CVD deaths (1961)*

Area as in Table V–4	Age groups 45—54 pop.	CVD	55—64 pop.	CVD	65—74 pop.	CVD	75 < pop.	CVD	40 < pop.	CVD	CVD*
A	184,948	36	146,378	159	93,376	389	48,242	733	567,294	1324	1264
B	82,584	18	67,250	54	46,193	219	25,737	533	264,660	827	790
C	6,310	0	5,205	7	3,645	11	1,972	49	20,243	67	68
D	17,551	7	15,219	14	10,829	48	6,052	118	58,403	187	201
E	54,296	15	44,739	32	30,174	128	17,516	382	173,449	558	606
F	94,303	16	77,183	79	52,756	259	27,320	579	299,961	934	939
G	63,692	17	51,219	48	33,226	153	16,890	397	198,164	621	588
H	66,037	16	53,044	65	34,389	199	17,379	364	205,348	645	617
I	28,256	7	23,659	36	13,823	61	8,228	164	85,240	268	252
Total	597,977	132	483,876	494	318,411	1467	169,336	3319	1872,762	5431	5325

* CVD deaths (total) for 1960

Table VI–a–1. *Age-adjusted average annual mortality rates, deaths per 100,000 population 1951—1958, for types of cerebrovascular disease*

Country	Type Subarachn. H (330)	Cb. H. (331)	Cb. Thr.-Emb. (332)	Other CVD (333—334)
Norway	2.3	46.2	4.7	44.7
Sweden	2.1	70.0	17.5	14.2
Denmark	1.3	70.0	17.4	10.8
Finland	5.2	100.6	37.2	9.5
Iceland	1.0	28.9	13.0	62.8
England-Wales	5.5	50.4	52.4	7.9
Scotland	3.3	69.9	65.6	9.3
Ireland	4.5	44.6	34.1	15.0
France	2.8	56.3	22.8	16.6
Netherlands	2.0	68.9	7.6	18.2
Belgium	0.5	14.3	22.8	10.7
Switzerland	1.5	20.5	6.4	80.7
Italy	1.0	53.3	44.6	26.2
Canada	2.7	55.9	25.8	12.2
USA (white)	2.9	59.6	23.0	9.3
Australia	4.5	58.9	44.0	10.6
New Zealand	6.0	43.2	43.1	9.2
U. So. Africa (white)	2.9	53.1	30.9	14.3
weighted mean	2.80	53.91	29.03	13.73

Table VI–a–2. *Subarachnoid hemorrhage vs. other CVD: Cumulative percent frequency by sex and type, CVD deaths in Denmark, 1956—1960*

Age	330 Subarachnoid			331—334 All others			330—334 Total		
	M	F	Σ	M	F	Σ	M	F	Σ
< 1	0.61	0.00	0.25	0.03	0.00	0.02	0.04	0.00	0.02
1— 4	0.61	0.84	0.75	0.03	0.01	0.03	0.04	0.03	0.04
5— 9	1.83	1.26	1.50	0.05	0.01	0.04	0.07	0.04	0.06
10—14	3.66	2.10	2.74	0.07	0.02	0.06	0.11	0.07	0.10
15—19	5.49	4.62	4.98	0.12	0.03	0.09	0.18	0.12	0.16
20—24	8.54	6.30	7.22	0.13	0.07	0.11	0.22	0.18	0.22
25—29	10.37	10.08	10.21	0.15	0.08	0.13	0.26	0.26	0.28
30—34	13.42	14.70	14.19	0.22	0.14	0.20	0.37	0.39	0.41
35—39	21.96	21.00	21.40	0.30	0.25	0.30	0.57	0.61	0.62
40—44	28.67	26.88	27.62	0.54	0.46	0.52	0.90	0.91	0.93
45—49	41.47	37.38	39.06	1.19	1.13	1.18	1.72	1.76	1.76
50—54	50.01	47.88	48.76	2.76	2.81	2.81	3.38	3.57	3.51
55—59	63.42	56.28	59.21	6.20	5.33	5.76	6.95	6.19	6.57
60—64	78.66	67.20	71.90	12.41	10.88	11.62	13.28	11.83	12.53
65—69	87.20	79.38	82.60	23.33	20.65	21.93	24.17	21.64	22.84
70—74	93.91	91.14	92.30	41.22	38.10	39.59	41.91	38.99	40.37
75—79	95.74	96.18	96.03	63.36	61.90	62.62	63.77	62.47	63.10
80 ≤	100.01	99.96	100.01	99.98	99.99	100.03	99.96	99.98	100.00
N	164	238	402	12,066	13,926	25,992	12,230	14,164	26,394
% Male	40.80			46.42			46.33		

Table VI-a-3. Average annual age-specific mortality rates, cases per 100,000 population, for Denmark, 1956—1960 for subarachnoid hemorrhage vs. other CVD with 95% confidence bands for the rates

Age	1958 pop. ×1000	Subarachnoid (330)			Other CVD (331—334)			Total CVD (330—334)		
		No. cases	rate obs.	range	No. cases	rate obs.	range	No. cases	rate obs.	range
0—14	1180.5	2.2	0.20	0.02— 0.64	2.6	0.22	0.04— 0.69	4.8	0.41	0.13— 0.96
15—19	338.9	1.8	0.53	0.06— 2.03	1.4	0.41	0.03— 1.84	3.2	0.94	0.21— 2.67
20—24	290.7	1.8	0.62	0.07— 2.37	1.2	0.41	0.02— 2.03	3.0	1.03	0.21— 3.02
25—29	278.6	2.4	0.86	0.13— 2.81	1.0	0.36	0.01— 2.00	3.4	1.22	0.29— 3.36
30—34	295.9	3.2	1.08	0.24— 3.06	3.4	1.15	0.27— 3.16	6.6	2.23	0.91— 4.69
35—39	313.1	5.8	1.85	0.66— 4.08	5.2	1.66	0.56— 3.82	11.0	3.51	1.76— 6.23
40—44	299.5	5.0	1.67	0.54— 3.90	11.6	3.87	1.98— 6.83	16.6	5.54	3.21— 8.92
45—49	309.4	9.2	2.97	1.38— 5.60	34.4	11.12	7.72— 15.51	43.6	14.09	10.22— 18.95
50—54	280.9	7.8	2.78	1.18— 5.55	84.6	30.12	24.05— 37.26	92.4	32.89	26.53— 39.94
55—59	249.7	8.4	3.36	1.49— 6.53	153.2	61.35	52.02— 71.87	161.6	64.72	55.13— 75.50
60—64	215.3	10.2	4.74	2.29— 8.66	304.4	141.38	125.95— 158.20	314.6	146.12	130.42— 163.20
65—69	170.7	8.6	5.04	2.26— 9.71	535.8	313.88	287.87— 341.63	544.4	318.92	292.69— 346.88
70—74	134.0	7.8	5.82	2.48—11.63	917.8	684.93	641.33— 730.71	925.6	690.75	646.96— 736.72
75—79	88.4	3.0	3.39	0.70— 9.92	1197.0	1354.07	1278.44—1433.00	1200.0	1357.47	1281.72—1436.50
80 ≤	69.5	3.2	4.60	1.02—13.04	1944.8	2798.27	2675.28—2925.44	1948.0	2802.88	2679.77—2930.14
Total	4515.1	80.4	1.78		5198.4	115.13		5278.8	116.91	

Table VI–a–4. *Average annual age-specific mortality rates for subarachnoid hemorrhage in the Netherlands, (A) 1950—1954, and (B) 1958—1962* (GIEL)

Age (A)	Population × 10 M			Cases			Annual rate per 100,000		
	M	F	Σ	M	F	Σ	M	F	Σ
0— 9	115	108	223	10	5	15	0.17	0.09	0.13
10—19	84	81	165	24	17	41	0.57	0.42	0.50
20—29	79	79	158	47	18	65	1.19	0.46	0.82
30—39	70	72	142	51	41	92	1.46	1.14	1.30
40—49	62	65	127	70	88	158	2.26	2.71	2.49
50—59	50	53	103	101	114	215	4.04	4.30	4.17
60 ≤	59	64	123	160	170	330	5.42	5.31	5.37
Σ	519	522	1041	463	453	916	1.78	1.74	1.76
				M/F ratio: 1.02			M/F ratio: 1.03		
(B)									
0— 9	116	110	226	12	3	15	0.21	0.05	0.13
10—19	109	104	213	25	23	48	0.46	0.44	0.45
20—29	80	78	158	53	34	87	1.33	0.87	1.10
30—39	75	77	152	81	56	137	2.16	1.45	1.80
40—49	66	69	135	123	132	255	3.73	3.83	3.78
50—59	58	62	120	141	201	342	4.86	6.48	5.70
60 ≤	72	81	153	259	312	571	7.19	7.70	7.46
Σ	576	581	1157	694	761	1455	2.41	2.62	2.52
				M/F ratio: 0.91			M/F ratio: 0.92		

Table VI–a–5. *Percentage frequency distribution by major causes, age, and sex for patients with first subarachnoid hemorrhage, from the Cooperative Study* (LOCKSLEY)

Age	Aneurysm			A-V malformation			Total*		
	M	F	Σ	M	F	Σ	M	F	Σ
0—14	0.7	0.4	0.5	8.2	2.4	5.5	1.7	0.6	1.1
15—24	5.5	1.3	3.0	16.3	20.8	18.4	5.3	2.5	3.8
25—34	11.2	3.9	6.9	20.4	24.8	22.4	9.9	5.5	7.5
35—44	23.0	14.3	17.8	18.4	21.6	19.9	18.4	13.3	15.7
45—54	33.1	27.1	29.5	19.0	15.2	17.3	29.6	24.3	26.8
55—64	20.6	28.7	25.4	15.6	10.4	13.2	23.9	28.1	26.2
65—74	5.4	19.7	13.8	2.0	4.8	3.3	9.0	19.1	14.5
75—84	0.5	4.3	2.7	—	—	—	2.0	5.7	4.0
85 ≤	—	0.3	0.2	—	—	—	0.2	0.8	0.5
Total	100.0	100.0	99.8	99.9	100.0	100.0	100.0	99.9	100.1
N	1086	1541	2627	147	125	272	2230	2650	4880
mean age	46.8	55.5	51.8	37.8	37.7	37.8	48.8	55.2	52.3
M/F ratio			0.70			1.18			0.84

* Includes 1981 "other" SAH

Table VI–a–6. *Age-distribution, cerebral aneurysms with subarachnoid hemorrhage, vs. brain tumors in Maida Vale Hospital, 1948 to 1960, from* DU BOULAY

Age	aneurysm	brain tumor
0— 5	0	0.5
6—15	1.1	2.2
16—25	3.5	4.7
26—35	7.6	12.3
36—45	24.9	16.0
46—55	35.0	31.2
56—65	23.4	25.5
66—75	4.6	6.4
76—85	0	0.7
86 ≤	0	0.5
Total	100.1	100.0
N	197	407

Table VI–a–7. *Percentage frequency distribution by site and sex for single aneurysms from the Cooperative Study* (LOCKSLEY)

Site	Male	Female	Total	M/F ratio	R/L ratio
Internal Carotid	29.8	49.8	41.2	0.44	1.16
Post. Communic. region	18.8	29.7	25.0	0.47	1.25
Other int. car.	11.0	20.1	16.2	0.40	1.04
Anterior Cerebral	44.7	25.2	33.5	1.31	1.00
Ant. Communic. region	38.3	20.3	28.0	1.39	—
Other ant. Cb.	6.4	4.9	5.5	0.97	1.00
Middle Cerebral	19.1	20.3	19.8	0.70	1.30
main branch region	11.5	12.6	12.1	0.68	1.31
Other mid. Cb.	7.6	7.7	7.7	0.72	1.28
Post. Circuit	6.3	4.7	5.4	0.97	1.39
post. Cb.	1.0	0.7	0.8	1.00	1.00
basilar	3.7	2.3	2.9	1.20	—
vertebral	1.0	0.9	0.9	0.79	2.57
cerebellar	0.6	0.8	0.7	0.55	1.00
Total	99.9	100.0	99.9	0.74	1.19
N	1135	1537	2672		

Table VI–a–8. *Percentage frequency distribution for age of patients with arteriovenous malformations (AVM) from the Cooperative Study* (PERRET)

Age	SAH c̄ AVM	AVM s̄ SAH	Σ AVM
0—10	4.9	5.5	5.1
11—20	18.2	6.8	14.6
21—30	21.5	17.1	20.1
31—40	22.8	26.0	23.8
41—50	15.6	24.0	18.3
51—60	12.7	13.7	13.0
61—70	3.3	5.5	4.0
71—74	1.0	1.4	1.1
	100.0	100.0	100.0
N	307	146	453
mean age	33.7	38.1	35.1
M/F ratio	1.06	1.15	1.09

Table VI–a–9. *Percentage frequency distributions for age of patients with AVM from the Mayo Clinic* (SVEIN)

Age	SAH c̄ AVM	AVM s̄ SAH	Σ AVM
0— 9	14.0	13.3	13.7
10—19	24.0	22.2	23.2
20—29	16.0	40.0	27.4
30—39	22.0	17.8	20.0
40—49	20.0	2.2	11.6
50 ≤	4.0	4.4	4.2
	100.0	99.9	100.1
N	50	45	95
median age	28	24	25
mean age	—	—	25.5
M/F ratio	0.85	1.65	1.16

Table VI–a–10. *Percentage frequency distribution by age for SAH with hypertension and/or arteriosclerosis from the Cooperative Study* (LOCKSLEY)

Age	Hypertension autopsied	alive*	Hypert. + Art. autopsied	alive*	Arteriosclerosis autopsied	alive*
0—10	1.3	—	—	—	—	—
11—20	—	—	—	—	—	—
21—30	2.6	—	1.5	—	—	6.7
31 40	3.8	8.0	5.9	—	2.4	—
41—50	20.5	29.3	17.6	5.9	12.2	20.0
51—60	33.3	38.7	25.5	47.1	19.5	46.7
61—70	24.4	21.3	32.4	35.3	22.0	20.0
71—80	12.8	2.7	12.7	5.9	26.8	6.7
81 ≤	1.3	—	4.4	5.9	17.1	—
Total	100.0	100.0	100.0	100.1	100.0	100.1
N	78	75	204	17	41	15
mean age	56.7	53.6	59.3	61.6	66.8	54.9
M/F ratio	1.05	0.60	1.17	1.43	1.41	1.14

* Alive at 90 days or more

Table VI–a–11. *Percentage frequency distribution by age for "idiopathic" SAH (no known associated disease) from the Cooperative Study* (LOCKSLEY)

Age	Autopsied	Alive*
0—10	—	1.0
11—20	3.2	3.5
21—30	6.5	7.0
31—40	14.5	12.6
41—50	17.7	25.2
51—60	16.1	32.9
61—70	19.4	17.1
71—80	14.5	0.7
81 ≤	8.1	—
Total	100.0	100.0
N	62	286
Mean age	55.0	48.3
MF/ratio	1.70	1.04

* Alive at 90 days or more

Table VI–a–13. *Male/Female ratios from sex and age-specific average annual mortality rates due to SAH in Denmark, 1956—1960*

Age	M/F	No. cases
15—19	0.49	9
20—24	1.24	9
25—29	0.34	12
30—34	0.47	16
35—39	0.96	29
40—44	0.81	25
45—49	0.86	46
50—54	0.58	39
55—59	1.19	42
60—64	1.07	51
65—69	0.55	43
70—74	0.45	39
75—79	0.29	15
80 ≤	0.92	16
Total	0.70	

N = 402

0 to 14 total =
11 cases in 5 years

Table VI–a–12. *Sex ratios for types of CVD: A. Subarachnoid hemorrhage (SAH)*

Source	Years	M/F (No.)	M/F (rates)	Med. age	N
I — Mortality statistics					
Denmark	1956—1960	0.69	0.70	55	402
England-Wales (DU BOULAY)	1960	0.61	—	57	3447
Surrey, England* (CRAWFORD)	1962—1963	1.17	1.18	—	78
Netherlands (GIEL)	1950—1954	1.02	1.03	54	916
Netherlands (GIEL)	1958—1962	0.91	0.92	55	1455
II — Hospital series					
London, Eng.* (DU BOULAY)	1948—1960	0.57	—	49	197
London, Eng.* (SARNER, 1967)	1958—1962	0.67	—	—	962
London, Eng.* (MCKISSOCK, 1964)	1952—1962	0.68	—	—	1686
Surrey, Eng.* (SARNER, 1965)	1962—1963	0.86	—	(all < 60)	106
Newcastle, Eng. (WALTON)	1940—1949	1.00	—	—	312
Rotterdam, Neth. (GIEL)	1951—1961	1.10	—	53	260
Rochester, Minn.* (UIHLEIN)	1957—1965	1.75	—	51	143
III — Population survey					
Surrey, Eng.* (CRAWFORD)	1962—1963	0.78	—	(all < 60)	57

* SAH due to aneurysm only

Table VII–a–1. Percent frequency by sex and type, CVD deaths in Denmark, 1956—1960, other than subarachnoid hemorrhage

Age	331 Cb. hemorrhage			332 Cb. thromb.-emb.			334 other			331—334 total		
	M	F	Σ	M	F	Σ	M	F	Σ	M	F	Σ
< 1	0.04	0	0.02	0	0	0	0.07	0	0.04	0.03	0	0.02
1— 4	0	0.01	0.01	0	0.04	0.02	0	0	0	0	0.01	0.01
5— 9	0.01	0	0.01	0	0	0	0.07	0	0.04	0.02	0	0.01
10—14	0.04	0.02	0.03	0	0	0	0	0	0	0.02	0.01	0.02
15—19	0.05	0.01	0.03	0	0	0	0.15	0	0.07	0.05	0.01	0.03
20—24	0.01	0.05	0.03	0	0	0	0	0	0	0.01	0.04	0.02
25—29	0.04	0.02	0.03	0	0	0	0	0	0	0.02	0.01	0.02
30—34	0.10	0.06	0.08	0.04	0.04	0.04	0	0.07	0.04	0.07	0.06	0.07
35—39	0.05	0.14	0.10	0.17	0	0.08	0.15	0.15	0.15	0.08	0.11	0.10
40—44	0.28	0.23	0.25	0.21	0.16	0.18	0.07	0.15	0.11	0.24	0.21	0.22
45—49	0.66	0.80	0.72	0.76	0.51	0.63	0.44	0.15	0.29	0.65	0.67	0.66
50—54	1.69	2.01	1.87	1.68	0.95	1.30	0.59	0.59	0.59	1.57	1.68	1.63
55—59	3.71	2.77	3.20	3.40	1.97	2.66	1.85	1.69	1.77	3.44	2.52	2.95
60—64	6.38	5.96	6.15	6.59	5.28	5.91	4.50	3.01	3.75	6.21	5.55	5.86
65—69	11.37	10.28	10.78	11.49	9.66	10.55	7.16	6.24	6.70	10.92	9.77	10.31
70—74	18.06	17.62	17.82	18.88	18.57	18.72	15.13	14.10	14.61	17.89	17.45	17.66
75—79	22.07	23.86	23.05	22.99	23.93	23.47	21.03	23.13	22.08	22.14	23.80	23.02
80 ≤	35.45	36.17	35.85	33.81	38.90	36.44	48.78	50.73	49.76	36.62	38.09	37.41
Σ	100.01	99.99	100.03	100.02	100.01	100.00	99.99	100.01	100.00	99.98	99.99	100.03
N	8327	10027	18354	2384	2537	4921	1355	1362	2717	12066	13926	25992
% Male	45.36			48.44			49.87			46.42		

Table VII–a–2. *Age-specific average annual mortality rates in cases per 100,000 population for types of CVD in Denmark, 1956—1960: cerebral hemorrhage (331); cerebral thrombosis-embolism (332); and other (334)*

Age	331 M	331 F	331 Σ	332 M	332 F	332 Σ	334 M	334 F	334 Σ
< 1	1.6	—	0.8	—	—	—	0.5	—	0.3
1— 4	—	0.1	0.1	—	0.1	0.1	—	—	—
5— 9	0.1	0.0	0.1	—	—	—	0.1	—	0.1
10—14	0.3	0.2	0.2	—	—	—	—	—	—
15—19	0.5	0.1	0.3	—	—	—	0.2	—	0.1
20—24	0.1	0.7	0.4	—	—	—	—	—	—
25—29	0.4	0.3	0.4	—	—	—	—	—	—
30—34	1.1	0.8	1.0	0.1	0.1	0.1	—	0.1	0.1
35—39	0.5	1.8	1.2	0.5	—	0.3	0.3	0.3	0.3
40—44	3.1	3.0	3.1	0.7	0.5	0.6	0.1	0.3	0.2
45—49	7.2	10.0	8.6	2.4	1.7	2.0	0.8	0.3	0.5
50—54	20.5	28.2	24.4	5.8	3.4	4.6	1.2	1.1	1.1
55—59	51.5	42.9	47.0	13.5	7.7	10.5	4.2	3.6	3.8
60—64	104.0	105.7	104.9	30.8	23.7	27.0	12.0	7.2	9.5
65—69	236.8	227.3	231.8	68.5	54.0	60.8	24.3	18.7	21.3
70—74	482.8	492.9	488.2	144.5	131.4	137.5	65.8	53.6	59.3
75—79	894.4	1011.4	957.0	266.7	256.7	261.3	138.7	133.2	135.8
80 ≤	1856.6	1924.1	1893.2	506.9	523.6	516.0	415.7	366.6	389.1
Total Annual Av.	74.4	88.1	81.3	21.3	22.3	21.8	12.1	12.0	12.0
No. cases	1665.4	2005.4	3670.8	476.8	507.4	984.2	271.0	272.4	543.4

Table VII–a–3. *Frequency distribution by percentage for A — cerebral thrombosis and other CVD, and B — cerebral hemorrhage, for cases from population surveys in USA*

Age group	A. — thrombosis and other (1) Middlesex	(2) Rochester	(3) Total	B. — hemorrhage (1) Middlesex	(2) Rochester	(3) Total
< 35	0	0	0	1.5	0	1.3
35—44	0.8	6.3	2.4	0	20	2.6
45—54	6.7	6.3	6.6	4.4	20	6.4
55—64	15.1	16.7	15.6	17.7	10	16.7
65—74	25.2	20.8	23.9	32.4	30	32.1
75—84	32.7	33.3	32.9	26.5	20	25.7
85 ≤	19.3	16.7	18.6	17.7	0	15.4
Total	99.8	100.1	100.0	100.2	100	100.2
N	119	48	167	68	10	78

Table VII−a−4. *Age-specific average annual mortality rates for cerebral hemorrhage in cases per 100,000 population for general hospital deaths in Göteborg, Sweden, (A) 1948—1949, and (B) 1960—1961* (AURELL)

Age	(A) 1948—1949			(B) 1960—1961			t*
	Population	No. cases	annual rate	Population	No. cases	annual rate	
30—39	61,225	5	4.08	50,813	0	0	1.58
40—49	54,678	6	5.49	61,592	4	3.25—	0.56
50—59	42,404	28	33.02	52,888	25	23.64	0.67
60—69	29,297	41	69.97	37,617	35	46.52	1.22
70—79	13,517	29	107.27	20,377	53	140.05—	0.06
80 ≤	3,495	11	157.37	5,667	34	299.98	0.01
Σ 30 ≤	204,616	120	29.32	228,954	149	32.54	0.60

* t = Test for significance of differences between respective mean rates

Table VII−a−5. *Age-specific annual incidence rates, cases per 100,000 population for cerebral hemorrhage from population surveys in USA*

Age	(1) Middlesex Conn.	(2) Rochester Minn.
< 35	2	0
35—44	0	40
45—54	30	50
55—64	160	30
65—74	380	130
75—84	680	170
85 ≤	1740	0
Average	60*	24
N	68	10

* Age-adjusted to US population

Table VII−a−6. *Sex ratios for types of CVD. B. Cerebral hemorrhage*

Source	Years	M/F (No.)	M/F (rates)	Med. age	N
I — Mortality statistics					
Denmark	1956—1960	0.83	0.84	78	18,354
England-Wales (DU BOULAY)	1960	0.68	—	—	28,991
II — Hospital series					
Vienna (FELGER)	1951—1955	1.34	—	53	138
Leipzig (ZIELKE)	1953—1961	0.68	—	66	372
III — Population survey					
Middlesex* (EISENBERG)	1957—1958	0.84	0.89	73	68

* Includes some cases of SAH

Table VII–a–7. *Male/Female ratios for sex and age-specific average annual mortality rates due to cerebral hemorrhage in Denmark, 1956—1960*

Age	M/F	N
15—19	3.83	5
20—24	0.20	6
25—29	1.57	5
30—34	1.38	14
35—39	0.29	18
40—44	1.02	46
45—49	0.72	133
50—54	0.72	343
55—59	1.20	587
60—64	0.98	1129
65—69	1.04	1978
70—74	0.98	3271
75—79	0.88	4230
80 $\leq$	0.96	6579
Total	0.84	
N		18354

0 to 14 total =
10 cases in 5 years

Table VII–a–8. *Percentage frequency distribution by age for recent encephalomalacia among 2650 autopsies in New Orleans* (Moossy, 1966)

Age	Male	Female	Total
30—39	1.3	3.0	2.1
40—49	7.9	9.1	8.5
50—59	21.3	16.7	19.0
60—69	28.9	27.3	28.2
70—79	25.0	33.3	28.9
80 $\leq$	15.8	10.6	13.4
	100.0	100.0	100.1
N	76	66	142 = 5.4 %
Median age	63	62	63

Table VII–a–9. *Age and sex specific rates in cases per 100 autopsies for occlusions of intracranial vessels among 4000 autopsies in New York* (Aronson)

Age	M	F	Total	N-(occlusions)	N-(autopsies)
16—25	—	—	—	0	78
26—35	1.2	1.0	1.1	2	191
36—45	2.0	2.7	2.3	9	387
46—55	5.1	6.3	5.6	35	625
56—65	7.3	7.4	7.3	61	832
66—75	6.9	8.4	7.6	73	967
76—85	7.5	10.5	9.0	65	721
86 $\leq$	7.1	4.3	5.4	11	202
Total	6.0	6.9	6.4		
N	130	126	256	256	4003
median age	—	—	—	69	64

Table VII−a−10. *Percentage frequency of compli-cated* intracranial arteriosclerotic changes and ence-phalomalacia by age among 122 adult autopsies in New Orleans* (MOOSSY, 1959)

Age	Compli-cated* arterio-sclerosis	Paren-chymal lesions	Number autop-sies
30—39	10	30	100=10
40—49	11	33	100= 9
50—59	21	33	100=24
60—69	13	39	100=23
70—79	32	50	100=22
80 ≤	33	56	100= 9
Total	16	32	100=
N	20	39	122

* Hemorrhage, thrombi, and/or calcium in plaque (*all* patients age 30 or more had cerebral arterio-sclerotic changes)

Table VII−a−11. *Relative frequency of thrombo-embolic occlusions by vessel in an autopsy series from Oslo* (JÖRGENSEN)

Locale	Percent (A)	Percent (B)	Percent (C)
Carotid	47.8	69.1	21.6
intracranial	24.8	35.7	18.9
extracranial	22.2	33.3	2.7
? primary site	0.9	—	—
Middle Cerebral	28.2	7.1	59.4
Ant. Cerebral	3.4	—	—
Basilar	4.3	2.4	10.8
Vertebral	6.0	9.5	—
Post. Inf. Cll.	1.7 ⎫ 9.4	⎫ 9.5	⎫ 8.1
Post. cerebral	7.7 ⎭	⎭	⎭
Subclavian	0.9	2.4	—
Total	100.0	100.0	100.0
N (lesions)	117	42	37
No. patients	101	37	33

(A) thromboembolic occlusions, total series, in 994 autopsies
(B) recent thrombotic occlusions *only*
(C) recent embolic occlusions *only*

Table VII–a–12. *Relative frequency of encephalo-malacia by region in an autopsy series* (ARONSON)

Region	N	Percentages Subtotal	Total
Frontal	507	24.8	19.3
Temporal	320	15.6	12.2
Parietal	364	17.8	13.8
Occipital	236	11.5	9.0
basal ganglia	621	30.3	23.6
Total cerebral	2048	100.0	77.9
Mid brain	45	14.8	1.7
Pons	244	80.0	9.3
Medulla	16	5.2	0.6
Total brain stem	305	100.0	11.6
Cerebellum	275	—	10.5
Total	2628*	—	100.0

* multiple lesions included (total autopsies, 4003)

Table VII–a–13. *Comparison of age distribution for carotid vs. basilar-vertebral thrombosis, from* McDOWELL

Age	carotid 0	E	basilar 0	E	total 0	E
<51	14	10.653	6	9.345	20	19.998
51—60	17	18.645	18	16.355	35	35.000
61—70	17	18.645	18	16.355	35	35.000
71≤	9	9.057	8	7.945	17	17.002
Total	57	57.000	50	50.000	107	107.000

$$\chi^2 = 2.869, \quad n = 3$$
$$0.5 > P > 0.3$$

t test for means: 58.98 vs. 61.60; t = 0.463; sex ratio: 68.4% vs. 66.0% male.

Table VII–a–14. *Frequency distribution by age, sex, and site for transient ischemic attacks (TIA) in London* (MARSHALL)

Age	carotid M	F	Σ	vertebrobasilar M	F	Σ	total* M	F	Σ
35—44	5.8	13.3	8.5	7.7	2.7	5.3	6.6	7.5	7.0
45—54	30.8	23.3	28.1	15.4	21.6	18.4	24.2	22.4	23.4
55—64	34.6	46.7	39.0	56.4	43.2	50.0	44.0	44.8	44.3
65—74	26.9	16.7	23.2	20.5	16.2	18.4	24.2	16.4	20.9
75—84	—	—	—	—	13.5	6.6	—	7.5	3.2
85≤	1.9	—	1.2	—	2.7	1.3	1.1	1.5	1.3
Σ (%)	100.0	100.0	100.0	100.0	99.9	100.0	100.1	100.1	100.1
N	52	30	82	39	37	76	91	67	158
Mean age	59.0	56.7	58.1	59.0	62.4	60.6	59.0	59.3	59.1
M/F ratio		1.73			1.05			1.36	

* Divided into three groups as of state when first seen: 68 with major CVA and history of prior TIA (Gp I); 61 with only TIA (Gp II); 29 with TIA only after major CVA (Gp III)

Table VII−a−15. *Sex ratios for types of CVD. C. Cerebral thrombosis-embolism*

Source	Years	M/F (No.)	M/F (rates)	Med. age	N
I — Mortality statistics					
Denmark	1956—1960	0.94	0.96	78	4,921
England-Wales (DU BOULAY)	1960	0.69	—	—	37,292
II — Hospital series					
Stockholm (LINDGREN)	to 1956	3.06	—	43	65
New York (MCDOWELL)	to 1960	2.06	—	60	107
Worcester, Mass. (ROBINSON)	1947—1956	0.84	—	69	933
London (MARSHALL, 1959)	c. 1958	2.22	—	58	177
Frederiksberg, Denmark (DALSGAARD)	1940—1953	0.73	—	c. 70	500
Leipzig (ZIELKE)	1953—1961	0.91	—	69	450
USA, 7 centers (FISHER)	1958—1959	1.72	—	(>55)	378
Middlesex, Eng. (CARTER)	1952—1961	1.04	—	65	612
III — Population surveys					
Framingham, Mass. (KANNEL)	1949—1962	0.90	1.13	59	57
Middlesex, Conn. (EISENBERG)	1957—1958	0.78	0.83	75	91
Goulburn, Australia (WALLACE)	1962—1964	0.91	—	69	450

Table VII−a−16. *Male/Female ratios for sex- and age-specific average annual mortality rates due to (1) cerebral thrombosis-embolism (332) and (2) other CVD (334) in Denmark, 1956—1960*

Age	332 M/F	N	334 M/F	N
40—44	1.28	9	0.54	3
45—49	1.41	31	3.00	8
50—54	1.74	64	1.04	16
55—59	1.75	131	1.18	48
60—64	1.30	291	1.65	102
65—69	1.27	519	1.29	182
70—74	1.10	921	1.23	397
75—79	1.04	1155	1.04	600
80 ≤	0.97	1793	1.13	1352
Total	0.96	4921	1.01	2717

0—39 total: 7 cases in 5 years; 9 cases in 5 years.

Table VII – a – 17. *Sex ratios for subdivisions of cerebral thrombosis-embolism*

Type	Years	M/F (No.)	M/F (rate)	Med. age	N
I — Autopsy data					
intracranial occlusion (1)	1958—1963	1.03	0.87*	68	256
encephalomalacia (1)	1958—1963	1.09	0.92*	69	2628
cerebral thrombosis (2)	1959	1.24	—	76	170
cerebral embolism (2)	1959	0.81	—	74	78
II — Hospital series					
carotid occlusion (3)	to 1956	3.00	—	43	40
carotid occlusion (4)	to 1960	2.16	—	60	57
basilar-vertebral occlusion (4)	to 1960	1.94	—	62	50
basilar-vertebral occlusion (5)	1958—1962	1.45	—	62	54
subclavian occlusion (6)	1962—1965	1.33	—	49	14
cerebral embolism (7)	1940—1953	0.42	—	—	68
cerebral embolism (8)	1940—1958	0.61	—	< 50	53

(1) ARONSON; (2) JÖRGENSEN; (3) LINDGREN; (4) McDOWELL; (5) BRADSHAW; (6) BRYANT; (7) DALSGAARD; (8) WELLS.

* Rates in cases per autopsies

Table VIII – a – 1. *Age and sex-specific annual mortality rates for CVD in non-whites of USA, 1960, in cases per 100,000 population*
(BERKSON)

Age	Male	Female
25—29	7.9	11.5
30—34	16.2	20.6
35—39	27.7	37.2
40—44	63.3	73.7
45—49	119.9	121.2
50—54	200.1	207.9
55—59	313.3	330.4
60—64	547.2	561.0
65—69	762.9	698.1
70—74	1024.2	964.0
75—79	1240.6	1211.2
80—84	1910.2	1768.8
85 ≤	2675.3	2510.2
Total (all ages)	118.2	121.2

Table VIII–a–2. *Estimated age and sex specific annual mortality rates for CVD in Negroes, 1960, using data of Table VIII–a–1, and population bias estimates* (SIRKEN)*

Age	Male		Female	
	Percent bias*	Corrected Rate	Percent bias*	Corrected Rate
25—29	+18	6.7	+ 6	10.8
30—34		13.7		19.4
35—39	+18	23.5—	+ 6	35.1
40—44		53.6		69.5
45—49	+26	95.2	+33	91.1
50—54		158.8		156.3
55—59	+32	237.3	+46	226.3
60—64		414.5		384.3
65—69	− 4	794.7	+11	628.9
70—74		1066.9		868.5—
75—79	−13	1426.0	− 4	1261.7
80—84		2195.6		1842.5
85 ≤	−22	3429.9	−10	2789.1

* Percentage deviation of observed from expected mortality rates, based upon the algebraic sum of similar deviations due to population undercounts and to age misreporting in mortality data (SIRKEN). See text.

Table VIII–a–3. *Cerebrovascular disease deaths in South Africa, 1954—1958, in cases per 100,000 population — age 40—74* (WALKER)

Age	White			Coloured*			Asiatic**		
	M	F	***	M	F	***	M	F	***
40—44	19.6	29.0	24.3	56.9	101.0	79.0	65.4	56.5	61.0
45—49	44.1	64.7	54.4	79.1	147.8	113.5	141.9	96.1	119.0
50—54	87.7	103.4	95.6	237.1	219.8	245.8	274.6	378.2	326.4
55—59	161.1	155.0	158.1	341.6	363.9	352.8	496.0	388.0	442.0
60—64	278.7	252.7	265.7	576.1	734.4	655.3	625.5	833.3	729.4
65—69	414.6	428.8	421.7	829.2	827.9	828.6	1059.2	1135.6	1097.4
70—74	657.2	734.3	695.8	1280.8	1145.1	1213.0	1806.3	2123.4	1964.9
Total population (all ages)	3 million			1.5 million			0.5 million		

* Coloured = part European (white) and African (Negro)
** Asiatic is almost entirely Indian
*** Unweighted mean

Table VIII−a−4. *Cerebrovascular disease deaths in Johannesburg, South Africa, expressed as percentage of total deaths for respective age, sex, and race; data for 1959—1960 for white and Bantu and 1955—1960 for Coloured and Asiatic* (WALKER)

Age	White		Coloured		Asiatic		Bantu	
	M	F	M	F	M	F	M	F
	percentages							
45—54	2.5 (13)*	5.2 (16)	4.2 (8)	8.4 (7)	7.2 (6)	5.2 (3)	4.9 (38)	9.3 (22)
55—64	3.1 (20)	5.0 (18)	11.6 (15)	9.4 (7)	9.4 (7)	13.4 (7)	2.5 (11)	7.4 (21)
65—74	3.3 (23)	6.1 (40)	6.4 (8)	10.5 (13)	10.0 (7)	15.8 (6)	6.8 (18)	6.1 (12)
75 ≤	6.2 (51)	7.5 (74)	10.3 (9)	11.6 (17)	9.4 (8)	15.0 (6)	8.2 (17)	8.6 (23)

Total population

(all ages)   376,000   40,000   28,000   594,000

* Number of CVD deaths in parentheses

Table VIII−a−5. *Cerebrovascular disease mortality rates in cases per 100,000 population for Japan, 1910*

Age	Male			Female			Total
	pop. ×1000	No.	rate	pop. ×1000	No.	rate	rate
0— 4	3165.1	268	8.5—	3076.9	217	7.1	7.8
5— 9	2882.0	66	2.3	2791.7	70	2.5	2.4
10—14	2556.8	52	2.0	2496.1	57	2.3	2.2
15—19	2252.0	87	3.9	2180.4	101	4.6	4.2
20—24	2089.5	140	6.7	2042.1	153	7.5	7.1
25—29	2003.7	260	13.0	1984.6	192	9.7	11.3
30—34	1875.3	423	22.6	1812.8	271	14.9	18.8
35—39	1473.9	648	44.0	1406.9	383	27.2	35.8
40—44	1445.1	1016	70.3	1363.0	715	52.5—	61.6
45—49	1114.5	1438	129.0	1061.5	918	86.5—	108.3
50—54	1176.7	2572	218.6	1121.5	1750	156.0	188.1
55—59	1008.0	3907	332.0	988.0	2678	271.1	329.9
60—64	801.7	5472	682.6	812.6	3877	477.1	579.1
65—69	550.7	6061	1100.6	593.1	4633	781.1	935.0
70—74	311.2	5168	1660.7	368.7	4754	1289.4	1459.1
75—79	198.9	4173	2098.0	255.4	4173	1633.9	1837.1
80—84	90.07	2078	2307.1	122.50	2462	2009.8	2135.8
85 ≤	49.54	762	1538.2	63.74	1037	1626.9	1588.1
Total	25,045.8	34,591	138.110	24,541.5	28,441	115.890	127.116

Table VIII−a−6. *Populations and cases of cerebral hemorrhage (331) by age and sex in Japan 1950 and 1962*

Age	1950 Male		Female		1962 Male		Female	
	pop. (m)	No.	pop. (m)	No.	pop. (m)	No.	pop. (m)	No.
0— 4	5718.5	38	5487.0	13	4000.	12	3838.	7
5— 9	4825.4	10	4697.2	13	4253.	10	4099.	1
10—14	4400.4	22	4299.5	19	5637.	15	5429.	9
15—19	4317.6	32	4250.1	28	4694.	19	4550.	11
20—24	3835.8	75	3889.7	48	4352.	27	4383.	31
25—29	2821.9	74	3363.2	73	4109.	71	4171.	41
30—34	2360.2	139	2842.0	134	3943.	249	3907.	82
35—39	2376.1	322	2672.0	382	3204.	435	3498.	237
40—44	2199.0	722	2284.0	791	2317.	887	2893.	562
45—49	2018.8	1571	1985.7	1632	2260.	1988	2609.	1378
50—54	1719.3	2834	1669.4	2722	2115.	4023	2350.	2798
55—59	1378.7	4274	1370.4	3641	1817.	6414	1856.	3810
60—64	1109.6	5897	1194.3	5170	1556.	9200	1640.	5634
65—69	795.9	7280	974.8	7309	1102.	11241	1225.	7815
70—74	540.3	7786	741.3	8520	745.	11487	914.	10112
75—79	267.7	5141	418.0	6768	400.	8832	585.	10202
80—84	95.6	2366	180.2	3657	179.	4749	328.	7301
85 ≤	28.8	816	66.7	1432	59.	1779	157.	3518
Total	40,811.8	39,409	42,387.9	42,362	46,744.	61,438	48,434.	53,549

Table VIII–a–7. *CVD Mortality in Japan — sex and age-specific rates in cases per 100,000 population. "Cerebral Hemorrhage" (331)*

Age	1950			1962		
	M	F	Σ	M	F	Σ
0— 4	0.7	0.2	0.5	0.3	0.2	0.2
5— 9	0.2	0.3	0.2	0.2	0.0	0.1
10—14	0.5	0.4	0.5	0.3	0.2	0.2
15—19	0.7	0.7	0.7	0.4	0.2	0.3
20—24	2.0	1.2	1.6	0.6	0.7	0.7
25—29	2.6	2.2	2.4	1.7	1.0	1.4
30—34	5.9	4.7	5.2	6.3	2.1	4.2
35—39	13.6	14.3	13.9	13.6	6.8	10.0
40—44	32.8	34.6	33.8	38.3	19.4	27.8
45—49	77.8	82.2	80.0	88.0	52.8	69.1
50—54	164.8	163.1	164.0	190.2	119.1	152.8
55—59	310.0	265.7	287.9	353.0	205.3	278.3
60—64	531.5	432.9	480.4	591.3	343.5	464.1
65—69	914.7	749.8	823.9	1020.1	638.0	818.9
70—74	1441.1	1149.3	1272.3	1541.9	1106.3	1301.9
75—79	1920.4	1619.1	1736.8	2208.0	1743.9	1934.4
80—84	2474.9	2029.4	2183.8	2653.1	2225.9	2372.0
85 ≤	2833.3	2146.9	2356.4	3015.3	2240.8	2452.3
Σ	96.56	99.94	98.28	131.44	110.56	120.81
N	39,409	42,362	81,771	61,438	53,549	114,987
pop. (× 1000)	40,811.8	42,387.9	83,199.6	46,744.	48,434.	95,178.
% CVD	92.36	92.59	92.48	71.54	71.07	71.32

Table VIII−a−8. *CVD Mortality in Japan — sex and age-specific rates in cases per 100,000 population: S.A.H. (330)*

Age	1950			1962		
	M	F	Σ	M	F	Σ
0— 4	0.2	0.2	0.2	0.3	0.2	0.2
5— 9	0.3	0.3	0.3	0.0	0.1	0.1
10—14	0.3	0.2	0.3	0.3	0.2	0.3
15—19	0.3	0.5	0.4	0.5	0.3	0.4
20—24	0.8	0.5	0.6	0.8	0.5	0.6
25—29	1.2	0.6	0.9	1.3	0.6	0.9
30—34	1.3	0.9	1.1	2.4	1.4	1.9
35—39	1.4	1.8	1.6	3.6	1.3	2.4
40—44	2.5	2.4	2.5	5.1	3.2	4.0
45—49	4.3	3.7	4.0	7.7	5.9	6.7
50—54	4.0	5.6	4.8	12.7	8.7	10.6
55—59	6.6	5.3	5.9	15.2	10.9	13.1
60—64	5.2	7.2	6.3	16.4	16.2	16.3
65—69	6.8	8.9	8.0	18.6	18.8	18.7
70—74	5.7	8.9	7.6	22.1	27.4	25.0
75—79	5.6	6.5	6.1	21.3	23.9	22.9
80—84	8.4	7.8	8.0	28.5	18.9	22.2
85 ≤	6.9	6.0	6.3	39.0	19.1	24.5
Σ	1.58	1.76	1.67	4.22	3.74	3.97
N	644	745	1389	1972	1810	3782
pop. (× 1000)	40,811.8	42,387.9	83,199.6	46,744.	48,434.	95,178.
% CVD	1.51	1.63	1.57	2.30	2.40	2.35

Table VIII–a–9. *CVD Mortality in Japan — sex and age-specific rates in cases per 100,000 population. "Cerebral thrombosis-embolism" (332)*

Age	1950			1962		
	M	F	Σ	M	F	Σ
0— 4	0.2	0.5	0.4	0.1	0.1	0.1
5— 9	0.2	0.2	0.2	0.1	0.1	0.1
10—14	0.2	0.2	0.2	0.1	0.1	0.1
15—19	0.3	0.5	0.4	0.4	0.3	0.3
20—24	0.8	0.8	0.8	0.4	0.5	0.4
25—29	1.3	1.1	1.2	0.4	0.7	0.5
30—34	1.4	1.3	1.4	1.0	1.0	1.0
35—39	1.3	2.1	1.7	1.4	1.7	1.6
40—44	1.6	2.1	1.9	2.7	3.0	2.9
45—49	3.1	3.7	3.4	5.5	5.9	5.7
50—54	4.6	6.4	5.5	15.9	13.4	14.6
55—59	9.9	7.7	8.8	42.9	27.4	35.0
60—64	18.9	13.0	15.8	97.9	55.9	76.3
65—69	28.5	21.4	24.6	213.3	130.4	169.7
70—74	51.5	30.1	39.1	413.4	267.6	333.1
75—79	76.2	36.8	52.2	447.3	386.0	411.3
80—84	78.5	73.8	75.4	388.3	337.8	354.9
85 ≤	111.1	75.0	86.0	201.7	166.2	175.9
Σ	3.78	3.45	3.61	29.93	26.44	28.16
N	1543	1462	3005	13990	12808	26798
pop. (× 1000)	40,811.8	42,387.9	83,199.6	46,744.	48,434.	95,178.
% CVD	3.62	3.20	3.40	16.29	17.00	16.62

Table VIII–a–10. *CVD Mortality in Japan — sex and age-specific rates in cases per 100,000 population. "Other and ill-defined conditions" (334)*

Age	1950			1962		
	M	F	Σ	M	F	Σ
0— 4	0.1	0.1	0.1	0.1	0.1	0.1
5— 9	0.1	0.0	0.1	0.0	—	0.0
10—14	0.0	0.0	0.0	—	0.0	0.0
15—19	—	0.1	0.0	0.1	0.0	0.1
20—24	0.1	0.1	0.1	0.2	0.1	0.1
25—29	0.1	0.1	0.1	0.3	0.3	0.3
30—34	0.3	0.1	0.2	0.6	0.4	0.5
35—39	0.5	0.2	0.3	1.5	0.5	1.0
40—44	0.5	0.7	0.6	3.5	1.6	2.4
45—49	1.2	1.3	1.2	9.5	5.1	7.1
50—54	2.7	1.9	2.3	20.8	12.6	16.5
55—59	5.0	6.2	5.6	42.4	23.2	32.7
60—64	12.9	10.1	11.5	76.0	40.3	57.7
65—69	28.0	20.7	24.0	128.1	75.3	100.3
70—74	42.8	36.0	38.9	225.1	147.4	182.3
75—79	60.5	49.3	53.7	349.8	251.3	291.6
80—84	80.5	76.0	77.6	457.5	345.1	384.1
85 ≤	142.4	93.0	108.0	600.0	426.8	474.1
Σ	2.59	2.78	2.69	18.08	14.79	16.41
N	1059	1177	2236	8453	7163	15,616
pop. (× 1000)	40,811.8	42,387.9	83,199.6	46,744.	48,434.	95,178.
% CVD	2.48	2.57	2.53	9.84	9.51	9.69

Table VIII–a–11. *CVD Mortality in Japan — sex and age-specific rates in cases per 100,000 population. "Cerebral thrombosis, embolism, and ill-defined" (332 + 334)*

Age	1950			1962		
	M	F	Σ	M	F	Σ
0— 4	0.3	0.6	0.4	0.2	0.2	0.2
5— 9	0.3	0.2	0.3	0.1	0.1	0.1
10—14	0.2	0.3	0.3	0.1	0.1	0.1
15—19	0.3	0.6	0.4	0.6	0.3	0.4
20—24	0.9	0.9	0.9	0.5	0.6	0.5
25—29	1.4	1.2	1.3	0.7	1.0	0.8
30—34	1.7	1.4	1.5	1.6	1.4	1.5
35—39	1.8	2.3	2.1	2.9	2.2	2.6
40—44	2.0	2.8	2.4	6.3	4.6	5.3
45—49	4.3	5.0	4.6	15.0	10.9	12.8
50—54	7.3	8.2	7.8	36.7	26.0	31.1
55—59	14.9	13.9	14.4	85.3	50.6	67.7
60—64	31.8	23.1	27.3	173.9	96.2	134.0
65—69	56.5	42.2	48.6	341.5	205.8	270.0
70—74	94.2	66.1	78.0	638.5	415.0	515.4
75—79	136.7	86.1	105.9	797.0	637.3	702.8
80—84	159.0	149.8	153.0	845.8	682.9	739.0
85 ≤	253.5	167.9	193.9	801.7	593.0	650.0
Σ	6.38	6.23	6.30	48.01	41.23	44.56
N	2602	2639	5241	22,443	19,971	42,414
pop. (× 1000)	40,811.8	42,387.9	83,199.6	46,744.	48,434.	95,178.
% CVD	6.10	5.77	5.93	26.13	26.51	26.31

Table VIII–a–12. *CVD mortality — Japan — sex and age-specific rates in cases per 100,000 population*

| Age | Total (330—334) | | | | | |
| | 1950 | | | 1962 | | |
	M	F	Σ	M	F	Σ
0— 4	1.1	1.1	1.1	0.8	0.5	0.7
5— 9	0.8	0.7	0.8	0.4	0.2	0.3
10—14	1.0	0.9	1.0	0.7	0.5	0.6
15—19	1.4	1.8	1.6	1.5	0.8	1.2
20—24	3.6	2.6	3.1	1.8	1.9	1.9
25—29	5.2	3.9	4.5	3.7	2.6	3.1
30—34	8.9	7.0	7.8	10.3	4.9	7.6
35—39	16.8	18.4	17.7	20.0	10.3	15.0
40—44	37.4	39.8	38.6	49.6	27.2	37.2
45—49	86.4	91.0	88.7	110.7	69.6	88.7
50—54	177.7	175.3	176.5	239.7	153.7	194.5
55—59	331.6	284.8	308.3	453.8	266.8	359.2
60—64	568.7	463.3	514.0	781.7	456.0	614.6
65—69	978.6	801.1	880.9	1380.3	862.7	1107.8
70—74	1541.2	1244.5	1358.0	2202.8	1548.9	1842.6
75—79	2063.5	1711.7	1849.1	3324.8	2529.7	2855.5
80—84	2642.3	2187.0	2344.8	4139.1	3279.9	3576.2
85 ≤	3093.8	2320.8	2556.6	5033.9	3561.1	3963.4
Σ	104.5	107.9	106.3	183.7	155.6	169.4
N	42668	45752	88420	85877	75351	161228
pop. (× 1000)	40,811.8	42,387.9	83,199.6	46,744.	48,434.	95,178.

Table VIII–a–13. *Diagnostic revisions with time for CVD in the first two years of the Hisayama study*

| Period:
Source: | 11/61—4/63
KATSUKI [1964 (1)] | | | 11/61—10/63
KATSUKI [1964 (2)] | | | 11/61—10/63
KATSUKI [1966 (2)] | | |
CVD	N	d	(*)	N	d	(*)	N	d	(*)
Cb. H.	—	10	(6)	9	7	(4)	9	8	(5)
Cb. thr.	—	3	(2)	11	2	(1)	13	5	(4)
Cb. Emb.	—	?	(—)	?	1	(1)	1	1	(1)
SAH	—	2	(2)	2	2	(2)	2	2	(2)
other	— 4 or 5		(0)	6	3	(0)	3	3	(0)
Total	—	18 or 19	(10)	28	15	(8)	28	19	(12)

* = Autopsies

Table XI–a–1. *Distribution of deaths by intervals after the ictus for age at ictus in all cerebrovascular disease cases in Middlesex, Conn.*

*	duration (mos.)	age >65	65—74	75≤	Total
a	to 0.07	8	8	18	34
b	0.08—0.25	8	18	19	45
c	0.26—0.5	2	4	11	17
	0.6—1.0	0	3	9	12
d	1.1—6.0	4	2	14	20
	6.1—12.0	2	5	2	9
e	12.1—36.0	6	3	8	17
	36.1—60.0	0	4	5	9
	Total deaths	30	47	86	163
	Total alive	14	7	7	28
	Total cases	44	54	93	191

* Groups a–e used for testing

$\chi^2 = 8.185$, n = 8 (0.50> P> 0.30)

χ^2 (alive vs. dead) = 14.260, n = 2 (P < 0.001)

Table XI–a–2. *Cumulative case-fatality rates from first SAH of varied cause treated non-surgically, from the Cooperative Study* (Locksley)

time	Cumulative fatality rates Single aneurysm	Multiple aneurysm	AVM	"other" SAH
1 day	9.6	9.1	7.1	11.6
7 days	26.7	23.8	12.5	23.5
14 days	38.5	41.7	16.3	29.3
21 days	45.5	47.2	19.0	32.2
28 days	49.4	50.8	—	33.4
42 days	54.6	56.0	20.5	34.9
90 days	58.6	61.9	21.7	36.4
180 days	60.7	63.0	22.8	38.0
360 days	62.7	64.3	25.4	38.6
2 years	64.8	66.3	26.5	40.4
3 years	65.5	68.3	27.6	41.7
> 3 years	67.7	69.8	29.7	43.7
N = 100.0	830	252	185	681

Table XI–a–3. *Distribution of deaths by intervals after ictus for cerebral hemorrhage vs. thrombosis cases in Middlesex, Conn.*

*	duration (mos.)	Cb. Hem.	Cb. Thromb.	Total
a	to 0.07	19	7	26
b	0.08—0.25	21	22	43
c	0.26—0.5	11	5	16
	0.6—1.0	5	6	11
d	1.1—6.0	3	15	18
	6.1—12.0	0	6	6
e	12.1—36.0	3	12	15
	36.1—60.0	1	7	8
	Total deaths	63	80	143
	Total alive	5	15	20
	Total cases	68	95	163

* Groups a–e used for testing

$\chi^2 = 26.39$, n = 4 (P < 0.001)

χ^2_c (alive vs. dead) = 1.895, n = 1 (0.20 > P > 0.10)

Table XI–a–4. *Comparison of course for carotid vs. basilar-vertebral thrombosis, data from* McDowell *(1961)*

Course	carotid		basilar		total	
	0	E	0	E	0	E
d. < 1 mo.	14	11.719	8	10.280	22	21.999
d. 1—24 mo.	4	7.991	11	7.010	15	15.001
alive p. 24 mo.	39	37.289	31	32.710	70	69.999
Total	57	56.999	50	50.000	107	106.999

$\chi^2 = 5.381$, n = 2

0.10 > P > 0.05

Table XII – a – 1. *Percentage frequency age distribution of intracranial vascular occlusions and encephalo-malacia among 4000 adult autopsies in New York* (ARONSON)

Age	Occlusions	Encephalo-malacia*	Autopsies
16—25	0	0.4	1.9
26—35	0.8	1.4	4.8
36—45	3.5	4.0	9.7
46—55	13.7	10.6	15.6
56—65	23.8	21.3	20.8
66—75	28.5	30.8	24.2
76—85	25.4	25.4	18.0
86 $\leq$	4.3	6.1	5.0
Total	100.0	100.0	100.0
N	256 persons	2628 lesions	4003
		($^1/_4$ of all autopsies)	
		($^2/_3$ of cases multiple)	

* Multiple lesions counted separately

Table XII – a – 2. *Age- and sex-specific mortality rates for all causes of death combined in England and Wales, expressed as cases per 1000 population, for 1851 and 1951* (TAYLOR)

Age	1851		1951	
	Male	Female	Male	Female
0— 4	72.9	62.9	7.4	5.7
5— 9	8.7	8.6	0.7	0.5—
10—14	4.9	5.3	0.6	0.4
15—19	6.7	7.6	0.9	0.6
20—24	8.8	8.8	1.4	0.9
25—34	9.5—	10.0	1.6	1.3
35—44	12.3	11.9	2.9	2.3
45—54	17.9	15.2	8.6	5.3
55—64	30.3	26.8	24.1	13.1
65—74	63.9	58.5	59.1	37.0
75—84	140.3	128.1	136.9	105.4
85 $\leq$	287.5	272.7	318.2	264.2
Total	22.8	21.2	31.4	11.8

Subject Index

Italicized page numbers refer to Text Tables or Figures

Aging and Cerebrovascular disease (CVD) 109—112
— summary 124
Aneurysm (see also SAH) 53—56
— age distributions 53, *54*
— course 99—100, *58, 98, 99, 100*
— locations 53—56, *55*
— proportions 53, *53, 58*
— summary 116—118, 121, 122
Anticoagulants in CVD 103
Arteriosclerosis
— and CVD 84
— autopsy data 63—64, 84
— epidemiology 83—84
— summary 120—121
Arteriovenous malformation (AVM) (see also SAH) 56—57
— clinical features 56—57, *53, 55, 58*
— course—99—101, *58, 98, 99*
— summary 117, 122
Associated factors in CVD 81—89
— conclusions 109
— summary 120—121

Cadmium and CVD 87
Calcium and CVD 87—88
Case-fatality rate, definition 2
Cerebral Embolism (see also Cb. Thromboembolism) 64—66, *65*
— summary 118
— treatment 103
Cerebral Hemorrhage 60—62
— changes with time 91—94, *91, 92*
— course 101, *101, 102*
— mortality data 60—62, *61*
— proportion of CVD 48
— sex ratios 61
— summary 116, 118, 121—123
Cerebral Thromboembolism 62—68
— autopsy data 63—64
— changes with time 92—95, *92*
— clinical types (q.v.) 64—68, *64, 65, 66, 67*
— course 101—104, *102, 103*
— incidence data 60—63, *62*
— mortality data 60—62, *61*
— proportion of CVD 48
— sex ratios 68, *65, 66*

Cerebral Thromboembolism
— summary 118—119
— treatment 103—104
— — anticoagulants 103
— — hyperbaric oxygen 104
— — operation 103—104
— — other drugs 104
Cerebral Thrombosis (see also Cb. Thromboembolism)
— carotid vs. vertebrobasilar 63—64, *64, 65*
— thrombosis vs. embolism 64—66, *65*
Cerebrovascular Disease (CVD) (see also specific types and sources)
— changes with time 90—95
— — summary 121—122
— conclusions 106—112
— — summary 123—124
— definitions 8—11
— — clinical definitions 10—11
— — ISC classification 8—10
— — summary 113—114
— general features 17—28
— — summary 114—115
— major divisions 47—50
— — relative frequency 47—50, *48, 49, 50, 51*
— — summary 116—117
— sex ratios 27—28, *28*
— — conclusions 108
— — summary 115
CVD Incidence 23—27, *24, 25, 26, 27*
— Carlisle, Eng. 24, *26*
— English general practices 24, *26*
— Goulburn, Australia 26, *27*
— Middlesex, Conn. 23, *24, 25*
— Missouri 24, *26*
— Rochester, Minn. 23, *25*
CVD Mortality
— age-specific rates 18—23
— — Canada *21*
— — Denmark *19*
— — Eire *20*
— — England-Wales *18*
— — Norway *20*
— — San Francisco *22*
— — Sweden *20*
— — Unites States *18*

CVD Mortality
— international comparisons 17—23, *17, 23*
— intranational comparisons 29—46
— summary 114
— vs. total mortality 110—112, *110, 111*
Cholesterol and Lipids in CVD 84—85
Coronary Artery Disease
— and CVD 84
— epidemiology 83—84
— heredity 86
Course of CVD (see also types of CVD)
    96—105
— all CVD 96—98, *97, 98*
— summary 122—123

Diabetes Mellitus and CVD 86

Encephalomalacia
— localization 64
— age-distribution *110*
Endarterectomy, Carotid 103—104
Epidemiology 1—7
— case material sources 2—5
— definition 1
— methods 2
— summary 113

Geographic Distribution of CVD 29—46
— conclusions 107—109
— correlations with medical facilities in
    Scandinavia 36—38, *37, 46*
— correlations with physicians in United
    States 41—46, *40, 41, 42, 43, 44, 45*
— Denmark 34—36, *34, 35, 36, 37*
— international comparisons 17—23
— Ireland 38—39, *38, 39*
— Norway 33—34, *32, 33*
— summary 115—116
— Sweden 30—33, *30, 31, 32, 33*
— United States 39—46, *40, 42, 43*
Genetic factors in CVD 86—87

Hypertension 81—83
— and CVD (see also CVD types) 82—83
— epidemiology 81—82
— in Japan and U.S. 84
— treatment and CVD 83, 104

Incidence Rate, definition 2
International Statistical Classification
    (ISC) of CVD 8—10
— fourth & fifth revision 92
— sixth & seventh revision 8—10
— suggested new code 106—107
— summary 113, 123

Japan and CVD 75—80

Japan and CVD 75—80
— autopsy confirmation 78—80, *79, 80*
— conclusions 109
— mortality data 75—78, *74—78*
— population data 77—80, *78, 79*
— summary 120

Lead and CVD 87

Medical facilities and CVD
— Scandinavia 36—38, *37, 46*
— United States 41—46, *40—45*
Mortality Data
— CVD, international comparisons
    17—23
— CVD, intranational comparisons
    29—46
— CVD, proportions of deaths *23, 78*
— in Japan, 1900—1960 *75*
— summary 114
— validity 12—16
Mortality Rate, definition 2

"Other" CVD (ISC 334)
— proportion of CVD 48
— mortality data *61*

Prevalence Rate, definition 2

Race and CVD 69—80
— conclusions 109
— Hawaii 77
— Japan (see Japan and CVD) 75—80
— South Africa 74—75, *73*
— summary 119—120
— U.S. Negroes 69—74, *69, 70, 72*
— U.S., other non-whites 71—72, *72*

Serum Lipids — see Cholesterol
Smoking and CVD 85—86
Statistical Testing 5—7
— chi-square test 5—6
— confidence limits 5
— correlation coefficients 6—7
Subarachnoid Hemorrhage (SAH)
— aneurysm (q.v.)
— AVM (q.v.)
— causes other than aneurysm or AVM
    56—57, *53, 58*
— changes with time 90—91, *91*
— clinical types 52—59, *53, 58*
— conclusions 108—109
— course 98—101, *58, 98, 99, 100*
— fatality and intracerebral hemorrhage
    99—100, *99, 100*
— frequency 50—52
— idiopathic 57, *56, 58*

Subarachnoid Hemorrhage
— integration   57—58, *58*
— mortality data   50—51, *48—52*
— proportion of CVD   48, 49, *48*
— summary   117—118

Transient Ischemic Attacks (TIA) (see also
    Thromboembolism)   66—68, *65, 66, 67*
Treatment
— in aneurysm   100—101

Treatment
— in AVM   101
— in cerebral hemorrhage   83, 101
— in cerebral thromboembolism
    103—104
Twin Studies and Vascular Disease
    86—87, *86*

Water Supply and Vascular Disease
    87—88

Printing: Carl Ritter & Co., Wiesbaden